DRIVE

9 Ways to Motivate Your Kids to Achieve

Janine Walker Caffrey, EdD

Da Capo
LIFE
LONG

A Member of the Perseus Books Group

Design and production by Eclipse Publishing Services
Set in 12 point Adobe Garamond

Cataloging-in-Publication data for this book is available
from the Library of Congress.

First Da Capo Press edition 2008
ISBN 978-0-7382-1160-2
Published by Da Capo Press
A Member of the Perseus Books Group
www.dacapopress.com

Da Capo Press books are available at special discounts for bulk purchases in the United States by corporations, institutions, and other organizations. For more information, please contact the Special Markets Department at the Perseus Books Group, 2300 Chestnut Street, Suite 200, Philadelphia, PA 19103, or call (800) 810-4145, ext. 5000, or e-mail special.markets@perseusbooks.com.

1 2 3 4 5 6 7 8 9 —12 11 10 09 08

*For Drew Caffrey, an amazing husband
and even more amazing dad*

Contents

Acknowledgments ix

ONE Your Child's Future 1

TWO The Driving Test 23
How Motivated Is Your Child?

THREE 1–Be a Pathfinder 35
*Gather the Info That
Really Makes a Difference*

FOUR 2–Increase Risk 57
Take Away the Plastic Bubble

FIVE 3–Decrease Rewards 71
*Allow Life's Natural
Consequences to Take Hold*

SIX 4–Deschedule 91
*Encourage Joy, Imagination,
and Creativity*

SEVEN 5–Reduce Comfort 109
*Counteract the Immense
Abundance and Indulgence
of Our Culture*

EIGHT 6–Delay Gratification 127
*Resist the Quick Fixes of
the Lottery, Game Shows,
and Reality TV*

NINE 7–Encourage Accomplishment 141
*Create a Sense of Self through
True Achievement*

TEN 8–Control the Crowd 159
*Use Peers for Positive Influence
and Independence*

ELEVEN 9–Create a Sense of Purpose 175
Make Life Meaningful

TWELVE Put Your Child 193
in the Driver's Seat
Apply the Lessons of Drive

Index *215*

Acknowledgments

Thanks to the parents of Renaissance Academy for entrusting me with your children's education, and to the students of Renaissance Academy for inspiring this book. I want you to dream big and keep moving until your dreams become reality. Thanks to the amazing staff of Renaissance Academy who are constantly trying new things and making our great school even better.

I am deeply indebted to my agent, Wendy Keller, who believed in me from the very beginning and kept agreeing to look at just one more proposal until I got it just right. I continue to value your guidance and friendship. Before my editor Katie McHugh got her hands on this book, it was an unsolved Rubik's Cube. Somehow she moved all of the colors to their proper positions and made it all make sense. Thanks, Katie.

Thanks to my parents, Adele and Howard Walker III, for instilling drive in me. You have given me the courage to take risks and appreciation for the gift of each day. My deepest gratitude goes to my husband Drew and our now grown children, Alison and Daniel. They have been reading my work leading up to this final product for nearly five years. Each of them has a keen eye for detail, and offers important guidance with each edit. Although their feedback was invaluable, it has been the life we share together that is the most important part of this book. I could not have chosen a better parenting partner than Drew. Raising our children (even though they are now adults) continues to be his most important life's work and he has sacrificed greatly to do it the right way. Drew and I truly enjoy each moment we have with our children as they reach each stage in their development. I can't imagine life without them.

DR⬆VE

Your Child's Future

Picture this: your child, who recently turned twenty-six, is sitting on the sofa in your home, clicking mindlessly from channel to channel. He has friends over late at night who eat your food and wake you up. Sometimes he works at a local restaurant, and sometimes he doesn't. He really wants to figure out where his life is headed (or so he says), but when you try to point him in the right direction—like school or training or another job—he fails to follow through. He keeps telling you not to pressure him. You ask him what he wants out of life, and he insists he is fine and content where he is.

Yikes! This will not be *your* child. He will make something of himself and leave home at a reasonable age. He will want things, do things, be things. He will launch a career. He will make a difference in the world by contributing to society and perhaps raising a family of his own. He will turn his passions in life into true purpose. Right?

For the past twenty-five years or so, I have been a teacher or administrator in many different schools, both public and private. I have worked with rich and poor families, amazingly smart and not-quite-as-smart kids, in cities and suburbs and country settings. Although the schools have all looked a little different, the kids have been generally the same. The cultural trends and generational similarities transcend socioeconomic levels, geographic locations, and students' abilities.

I have noticed that many of today's kids have something in particular in common: a lack of personal drive. They don't seem to want things and are unaware of what life has to offer and how to get it. They seem to believe that things will be handed to them when needed and that life will be fine, with or without their effort and input. These young people are content to allow things to happen to them and drift along wherever life takes them.

Maria, twelve years old, was a very sweet child who never caused a problem. She was not unhappy and was perfectly content to sit on the couch for hours at a time, snacking and watching her favorite shows on TLC. Her mom constantly nagged her to get up and do something, taking her shopping at the mall, taking her to get her hair done, and even redecorating her room in an attempt to motivate her. But Maria didn't seem to want to do anything except watch TV or message her friends on MySpace. At her old school, Maria was absent at least once every week or two and didn't seem to care about anything. Her grades hovered somewhere between Bs and Ds, but she always seemed to just squeak by at the end of each grading period. This didn't seem to concern her; she thought she was getting by fine.

I see a lack of motivation like Maria's in many children. I began noticing this problem when my own son approached adolescence. Many of his friends lacked the motivation to do schoolwork, to participate in activities, or even to take field trips with school. As he moved through middle and high school, the problem became more and more pronounced. As an educator, I was acutely aware of the trend within the schools where I worked. We would announce a dance or an event, or even an overnight trip, and students would not sign up. They would say things like, "That doesn't interest me" or "I don't want to do that." They would miss opportunity after opportunity for no apparent reason. When I spoke with these students' parents, they would shy away from the problem, stating that they didn't want to force their children to do things. When I observed these same teens not wanting to drive their cars (which had often been given to them before they were of legal age to drive), I knew something was wrong. I began researching the issue and found it to be a very common problem that was baffling adolescent development experts across the country.

Often, though, parents tell me, "I'm sure his disinterest in life is only a phase. His fear of new things will certainly pass with age." However, if you are noticing that your child seems apathetic, time alone will not necessarily improve the situation.

This book will show you how to help your child gain a sense of accomplishment and surround himself with friends who do the same. Soon your child will learn how to overcome obstacles and move toward the goals he has set for himself. Whether in middle school, in high school, in college, or beyond, your child can develop the drive he needs to become successful and transform into an amazing, independent adult.

The Millennials: Generation Me

If your child was born between 1981 and 1996 or perhaps beyond, she is part of what is referred to as the "millennial generation." These young people, also known as Generation Me, often grew up as the center of their parents' universe and have been coddled, comforted, and revered, leading to several common attributes. Some of these traits are very positive, while others are not.

According to the Center for Generational Studies, our children have adapted remarkably to the modern world and have a firm grasp on the latest advancements in science and portable technology. Of course, you don't need a study to tell you this—chances are, you know how much your child loves to instant-message, check Facebook, text away on her cell phone, and hook up her iPod (and tune you out). However, this proclivity also means children tend to rely on the *immediacy* of such technology. Along with a sense of instant gratification, teens' affinity for technology makes them the ultimate consumers, which causes many of them to believe that the only purpose for earning money is to spend it on the latest—be it a gadget, handbag, or automobile.

Another trait of this generation is that they question everything—including authority and traditional conventions—much more so than children of previous generations.

The best place to see examples of this phenomenon is within romantic relationships. Decades ago, there were only a few different categories of relationships. You were either "going together" or not. You might live together or not, or get married or divorced. Recently, I was talking to a graduate of the school I founded (which will be discussed later). Imar is now twenty-one years old and living in Texas. She began talking about a young man named Robert. I asked her if he was her boyfriend. Her response, which I have heard more times than I can count from twentysomethings, was "It's complicated." When I asked what she meant by that, she started describing the many phases of their relationship that had occurred over the past several months. At times she had been "talking to" Robert. Other times she was "kinda seeing him" or "together" with him, but sometimes she was "hooking up" with another guy who was a "friend with benefits." She was thinking about living with Robert just to see what might happen but couldn't even think about what the future might hold.

While this questioning of conventions allows millennials to think in new ways, it also causes them to question themselves and the direction their life takes at every turn. They tend to learn to drive later, take longer to complete their education, live with their parents longer, marry later (if at all), have children outside of marriage at an ever increasing rate, and return home frequently.*

Throughout their childhood, millennial kids have been plugged into sports, youth groups, playdates, and other organized activities more than children before them. To be sure, these activities have positives—they offer lots of wonderful and diverse experiences. Too much structured activity, however, can rob kids of the ability to imagine and play in a way that comes naturally to them. As they grow, they continue to need a great deal of structure and must be given clear expectations every step of the way, even as adults.

The millennials have grown up in a culture that is safer than ever before. According to a 2005 report by the U.S. Department of Justice, 115 children were abducted by nonfamily members in 1999. Although just one would be too many, abductions are a very rare event. This data suggests a decline in kidnapping incidents, although many parents believe abductions are on the rise. According to the FBI's Uniform Crime Report from 2004, violent crimes in the United States decreased by an impressive 24 percent during the previous decade. Yet we live in a world of 24/7 media, thanks to the Internet and television, and due to increased media coverage of horrific events, we fear continually for our children's safety. In an effort to shield children from danger, parents sometimes unwittingly keep them from making mistakes and taking the risks that allow them to develop the competency and courage necessary for a full, rich life.

* Constance Alexander, "Each Generation Has its Themes," July, 2001, http://www .gentrends.com (accessed January, 2007).

⬆ Drive: The Generation Gap

The matures. The generation called "matures" includes people born before World War II. Most of them experienced the effects of the stock market crash of 1929 and the succeeding era known as the Great Depression. They understand what true poverty is, may remember not having enough food, and understand the value of hard work. This group tends to be thrifty, fast working, and intensely loyal. They are willing to sacrifice and delay gratification. From their perspective, employers and employees have a duty to one another. There is an inherent pessimism in this group because they experienced great loss during the Depression and World War II. The mature generation is driven by a *sense of survival.*

Baby boomers. After World War II, the baby boomer generation was born. This is the largest generational group in American history and has shaped much of our culture and commercially driven economy. This group is all about optimism, efficiency, having lots of credit to buy things now and pay later. As youth of the 1960s, they have had a history of being socially conscious. However, they have tended to become more conservative in their political views as they have moved into middle and senior age. They do not assume any loyalty between employer and employee because they experienced the layoffs and shortages prevalent in the 1970s. The baby boomer generation is driven by *wanting more than their parents had.*

Generation X. Children who were born in the mid to late 1960s through the early 1980s are collectively known as

Generation X. This group has witnessed the difficulties that come from overextending credit and are more apt to save. However, they tend to live for today in all other respects. They question the validity of tasks and find ways to eliminate any work they feel is unnecessary. Gen Xers are very focused on themselves and have more difficulty doing what is good for an entire group. They witnessed much uncertainty when they were growing up in the form of lost jobs, increasing divorce rates, and a shifting morality. Therefore, they tend to be a bit skeptical about opportunity and future plans. Generation X is driven by their *fear of the unknown.*

Millennial generation (Generation Y or Generation Me). Toward the end of the twentieth century, Generation Me was born. This group, now coming of age, tends to earn to spend. Their culture has been operating at warp speed, with new technology making it move faster all the time. They want what they want when they want it. This group tends to see their parents as friends and are much more connected to their families. At the same time, however, they lead very separate lives from the others living in their households. They are more likely to eat on the run and less likely to sit down to dinner with their parents. Parents, teachers, and others responsible for the care of Generation Me have done a great job of orchestrating every facet of their lives. This has led to their extreme need for structure and direction. This group needs to be told exactly what is expected of them as much as possible. Generation Me is *not driven* because they have wanted for little in a safe and predictable world.

The cumulative result of these factors is a generation of young people who tend to lack drive, the power to propel their lives forward.

Drive is what creates the fire in the belly to become an independent adult and get things done. It is what moves us and creates a force for achievement and change. Let's take a look at the life of an adult who is driven.

Driven to Success: Howard Schultz's Story

Haven't heard of Howard Schultz? Chances are you may experience a little of his influence every day.

Howard Schultz, a member of the baby boomer generation, was born in 1952 and raised in a housing project in Brooklyn. Like most kids in his neighborhood, he played in the streets, climbed trees, and engaged in what we might consider risky behavior today. There were no after-school programs, music lessons, or structured activities other than traditional school. Howard was often responsible for his younger brother, as he describes in his 1997 book, *Pour Your Heart into It*: "I was able to insulate my brother Robert from the economic hardship I felt and give him the kind of guidance my parents couldn't offer." Howard spent all his free time in pickup games in the schoolyard where hundreds of kids would compete for game time. "You had to be good there, because if you didn't win, you'd be out of the game, forced to watch for hours before you could get back in. So I played to win."

Howard's family didn't have much, so he did not get an allowance or many toys or other material goods. Anything that came their way was earned, over time, through hard work. In 1959, when Howard was seven, what little his family had was taken away suddenly when his father broke a leg and could no longer work as a delivery driver. The family had very little and struggled just to survive. In a *60 Minutes* interview aired on April 23, 2006, Howard described how this life event impacted him and made him dream of getting out of the projects: "I saw the plight of a working-class family, I saw the fracturing of the American dream firsthand at the age of seven. That memory scarred me."

Howard put himself through college, working at all kinds of jobs and even selling his own blood to earn money. It certainly seems as if Howard did not have many advantages or an easy time. But in hearing his story, I'd argue that Howard's very lack of a cocoon of safety, positive behavior plans, after-school programs, and affluence were the fuel that created his extreme drive.

As a young adult, Howard worked for a company that did business with Starbucks, then a small operation in Seattle. He was impressed with the organization and began working there. After a few years, he was offered a chance to buy Starbucks. He had a vision for the company and set out to make it happen. Many thought he was nuts.

As he asked in the interview on *60 Minutes*, "If I came to you in 1987 and I said to you, 'Even though coffee consumption in America is down, I wanna build a company that was gonna sell coffee not in a porcelain cup but in a paper cup, with Italian-sounding words that no one could pronounce, for three dollars a cup of coffee,' would you invest?"

So how was Howard Schultz able to get people to take that big of a risk with their money? Howard could see the vision for this company and had the tenacity—the drive—to keep going in his quest for investors. Drive is what allows us to conquer our fears. Drive is what keeps us moving toward a goal. Drive is the push that overcomes all obstacles. Watching Howard Schultz in action is watching drive in motion.

Starbucks is now an international company that creates culture and provides top benefits for its employees so that other families do not suffer the same fate as Howard Schultz's. Scott Pelley, in his *60 Minutes* story on Howard, stated, "Schultz has organized his company around that memory [of growing up poor]. He provides health insurance to employees who work as little as twenty hours a week. He raised prices to do it. And now Starbucks spends more on health care than it does on coffee."

The Realities of Modern American Life

Of course, I am not advocating that children grow up in poverty. But to truly understand drive, we need to examine the realities of modern American life and how they tend to impede our children's desire to move forward.

Dependency

Howard Schultz grew up long before children were given cell phones. He spent most of his day away from his parents, making decisions on his own and developing independence in the process. Today children are in constant communication with their parents. If there is a problem at school, parents sometimes know about it before the principal, thanks to cell phones. Children constantly seek their parents' guidance on mundane issues, seemingly unable to make a move without support. At a time in their lives when they should be developing independence, I see young people become even more dependent on their parents, continually questioning themselves and calling for advice.

Teens and young adults often find it difficult to manage the constant intrusions of cell phones and other electronic devices and find themselves distracted by friends and family when they should be studying or working or interacting with the people around them. All this communication makes it very challenging for a teen to do what comes naturally: to pull away from her parents. Cell phones are like an electronic umbilical chord that keeps a child connected through the college years and beyond. College students today report being on the phone with their parents sometimes several times a day. Some parents actually provide daily wake-up calls to their children and keep track of their children's schedules and homework! While this advent of technology can be helpful as parents begin to let go, it can also hinder the process. If a parent continues to hover, the child will not likely feel the need to separate and develop the skills necessary to lead her own life. People with drive are eager to assume their own lives and look forward to creating a home and identity separate from their parents.

In this book, you'll learn how to be an involved parent while still fostering your child's independence.

The Plastic Bubble

Bill Cosby has said on many occasions that you don't know fear until you become a parent. The round-the-clock media coverage amplifies our natural fears. We learn about every child who is missing or harmed and hear about such children continually until they are found, or as long as our attention is sustainable in the cases when they aren't found. There are toy and other product recalls and hidden dangers in just about everything. As our children grow, we become increasingly afraid that someone will harm them, take them, or kill them. Shopping malls host fingerprinting festivals, providing parents a record to identify their child in case she is taken from them. We constantly hear about freak accidents when children are killed by falling off a skateboard or jumping from a tree. Although our children are actually safer than they have ever been, we are so acutely aware of all the dangers, we tend to believe that they are more at risk than ever before.

One of the schools where I taught is an old-fashioned neighborhood school. All the elementary school children who attend live in that neighborhood, within a radius of about three quarters of a mile, an easy walk for most kids. Yet every day, immediately before and after school, a long line of cars forms to drop off and pick up children. Very few kids walk or ride bikes to school. I thought this was very strange, so I started asking the kids why they weren't walking or biking. They told me that their parents wouldn't allow them to walk or bike because they might get hurt. When I inquired further and followed up with the parents, I learned that these parents—who live in a very safe, upscale, suburban neighborhood—are worried about stranger abductions, biking accidents, unstable surfaces, cars, and so forth. They are convinced that their children are in real danger, so they choose to drive them to and from school. In their attempt to protect their children, they are depriving them of a wonderful opportunity to gain independence and confidence.

We must provide important experiences, with guidance and calculated risk, that develop these instincts while still keeping children safe. Children who are not completely protected from life tend to develop street smarts that cannot be taught. It is only through interacting with the world, and sometimes getting hurt, that young people learn to judge and anticipate true harm. In the long run, children who learn through these kinds of experiences are actually safer because they learn to keep themselves free from harm when their parents are not around. People with drive are not afraid of taking risks. They understand that failing makes them stronger and are willing to take chances to improve their lives.

Rewards without Consequences

Ever since Dr. Spock, American parents have turned to the popular psychologist of the day to assist them in raising their children. Just watch one of today's nanny television shows, and you will see complicated behavior charts that provide rewards for speaking respectfully to parents, sharing toys, and other examples of being good.

These same rewards are taken away when the child is naughty by doing things like talking back or stealing a sibling's toys. Many parents and teachers use these elaborate systems. But when a child's behavior is continually managed this way, good behavior is often overly rewarded, and bad behavior is often not directly addressed.

I know several parents who have instituted a toy-dollar system in their homes. They give their children points on a chart for certain behaviors and then convert the points into cash that can be used to buy toys. They go to the local toy store each weekend to allow their children, ranging in age from five to nine, to pick out a toy with their money. While on the surface this seems like a good idea, it tends to backfire. One day when I was visiting one of the toy-dollar families, I witnessed an exchange that illustrates beautifully the pitfalls of overrewarding. The mom asked her seven-year-old son to help his younger brother brush his teeth and hair. The seven-year-old looked at her intently for a few moments. You could tell he was working hard to formulate exactly the right words before speaking. Finally, he said, "How many toy dollars will I earn?" The mother didn't miss a beat in responding. She said, "Helping your brother is not on your toy-dollar chart." To which the young negotiator retorted, "Then we need to add it."

Now here is the truly amazing part. The mother quickly turned toward the fridge where the chart was hanging and added the behavior. She turned back to her boys and said, "That was a great idea. Helping your brother is worth one toy dollar."

While these reward systems are somewhat effective, children have become increasingly savvy and have learned to manipulate them to maximize rewards. This is particularly true for children with parents who may disagree about parenting strategies or who live apart. Children learn that they are in charge and do not learn to respect the authority of a parent, teacher, or other figure. They learn that they do things to get things, instead of doing the right things and simply respecting authority. People with drive do the things that need to be done without expecting rewards. Although they often have an entrepreneurial spirit, they understand how to work with authority to achieve success.

Overscheduled Activities

Gymboree. Baby sign language. Toddler music classes. Preschool sports. Swim lessons. Summer camps. Foreign language classes. Children are placed into all types of programs from almost the time they are born. We live in a wonderful world that provides many opportunities for our kids to grow and learn, and there's nothing inherently wrong with any of them—in fact, arts and athletics programs can be of real help to kids. But you can have too much of a good thing. Many young children now have all their play scheduled *for* them! It's hard to believe that there was a time when kids had to make their own fun through invented games and imaginative play. The "sports program" consisted of stickball in an alley or a pickup game of kickball in the backyard. "Summer camp" may have included a game of marbles or putting on a show, using old sheets for the curtain.

Cathy and Joe want their two children, Megan and Hayden, to experience everything so the kids might gain an edge over their peers. These parents also rely on the endless activities to serve as childcare so they can work or engage in their own activities. In an age when Americans have more leisure time than ever before, they find themselves busier than ever, racing constantly to the next thing and the next thing and the next. Every minute of every day is jammed with programs and activities designed to keep kids busy and allow moms and dads to do the things they need to do. Meals are often eaten on the run in the family van or SUV. The logistics of running Cathy and Joe's fairly typical household resemble complex military maneuvers to ensure everyone gets to the right place at the right time.

Cathy and Joe find themselves in a world where we all expect to be entertained as we wait. In the family vehicle is a DVD player to mesmerize the children as they are chauffeured throughout the community. In the doctor's office, the grocery checkout, the post office, and any other place where they wait are televisions designed to distract them to make the wait seem shorter. Megan's and Hayden's bedrooms are electronics amusement parks with visual, auditory, and kinesthetic stimuli for every mood. As a result, Megan and Hayden have no idea how to use their time. They have forgotten how to pretend, how to dream, how to make their own fun. The moment there is more than a few moments of unoccupied time, they proclaim, "I'm *bored*!" When this happens, Cathy or Joe quickly comes to the rescue with some activity designed to distract and entertain.

David Elkind, PhD, has become an advocate to preserve childhood and allow children to learn by doing what comes naturally to them. In his book *The Power of Play*, Dr. Elkind uses child development research to help parents understand the true advantages a child will have from a less structured schedule. A child who is never afforded the opportunity to use his own time to create and imagine is constantly in need of being entertained—relying on external, rather than internal, motivation. People with drive use their time to fuel their passions by envisioning a future full of wonderful expectations.

Abundance

Americans live in an era of unprecedented affluence. Although many families feel as if they have less than before, they actually have more than any other generation before them. Consider the size of our homes and the amount of stuff—clothes, toys, gadgets, furniture—in those homes. Many families need to rent storage spaces just to keep it all. Consider the number, age, and value of our automobiles. Consider the amount of disposable income spent on movies, candy, diversions, and the other joys of life. Compare these to what our parents and grandparents had.

What does your child have in his room? Expensive electronics? Closets full of designer clothes? His own phone? Hundreds of toys? A typical American child has more luxuries in his own room than entire families had in the 1950s and 1960s. The problem is that many kids come to believe they are entitled to all these things. They think that they should be able to have whatever they want whenever they want. They live in an age when meals come with toys, when most eleven-year-olds have cell phones, and when a car is bestowed on every teen who reaches driving age. This has created huge stress for children and adults. Young adults are sadder than ever as a result of this dichotomy. Jean Twenge, PhD, chronicled this phenomenon in her 2006 book, *Generation Me: Why Today's Young Americans Are More Confident, Assertive, Entitled—and More Miserable Than Ever Before*. Young adults expect when they begin their lives independent of their parents that they will magically continue to get all the things they had as children. Unfortunately, this is not the case. When reality does not meet their expectations, they quickly become frustrated and experience what is now referred to as a "quarterlife crisis." * Many end up moving back into their parents' homes (if they moved out in the first place) in response to their disappointment. Having more has actually caused many young people to believe they don't have enough.

A great example of this can be seen with teens and their cars. In my community, nearly all parents give their children a car. It seems that a vehicle has now become a necessity, not a luxury, for our youngest drivers. I had one student who was given *three* cars. He

---

* Alexandra Robbins and Abby Wilner, *The Quarterlife Crisis* (New York: Penguin Putnam Books, 2001).

got one a full year before he received his driver's license and two more when he crashed what he had. Yet this teen always felt that he was poor. He constantly complained that other kids had nicer cars and couldn't understand why his parents wouldn't give him what he felt he deserved. He was miserable most of the time, always focusing on the new BMW or Volvo that another student had received.

Growing up with great abundance can create a false security and expectation that children should have whatever they desire at all times, rather than an understanding that to get the things they want, they need to work hard.

Immediate Gratification

The poor souls who audition for *American Idol* and don't make the cut are crushed. "This was my only chance to make it," some will say. "They just don't understand my talent," say others after tone-deaf auditions. There are sad tales of woe from those who have quit their jobs or taken time off from school to make the trip. It is not uncommon for a wannabe to proclaim, "But I am supposed to be famous!" This is one very visible example of our fixation with immediate gratification. Reality television is full of stories of people winning new homes, trips, and even spouses. The proliferation of lotteries and gaming has increased Americans' obsession for gambling and belief that their lives can be transformed overnight. Families receive a constant flow of new credit card offers in the mail—sending the message that you can always buy more, even if you don't have the money.

By teaching kids that they need to wait for things of value and work hard for what they have—by encouraging them to earn good grades and save money over time—you can help your children develop that fire in the belly that will move them to create and push and grind and scrape to make things happen. People with drive are able to delay gratification and work toward long-term goals that really matter.

Underachievement

Self-esteem is great. The better we feel about ourselves, the more successful we are sure to become. But in some ways, we may have taken it too far. The self-esteem movement of the 1980s and 1990s created programs, gimmicks, therapies, strategies, and even courses designed to make kids feel good about themselves. Self-esteem was linked to every conceivable advantage of life. We all believed that if children were told how special they were, they would somehow transform into high-achieving, wealthy, happy adults. While it is true that there is a link between self-esteem and success, it seems that we got the order of the association wrong. We develop actual self-esteem *because* we are successful, not the other way around. True achievement is its own reward.

When I was in college in the early 1980s, studying to be a teacher, my peers and I were actually taught to reward nonachievement. It was drilled into our heads in many of our classes that we needed to praise and reward at every opportunity. If students play a game in class, the teacher should give every player a prize just for participating. If a school or class gives awards at the end of the year, we were taught to come up with an award for every single student. We were taught to have a full arsenal of stickers, trinkets, and other fun items to give to our kids daily so they would always feel good about themselves. In one class, the professor actually had us learn a full menu of chants that we could teach children of all ages to help reinforce how special they were.

Rewarding everything—which may or may not include real achievement—actually robs children (and adults) of the motivation to succeed. If everyone is rewarded the same regardless of effort or success, why would one strive to do more? In an effort to minimize the negative effects of competition, we have eliminated many of its positive effects. Children need a healthy balance of opportunities to stretch, grow, and compete to develop the drive they need for success. People with drive love to compete and understand that it makes them stronger and better.

The School of Drive

As an educator, my concerns about the lack of motivation I was seeing in kids grew so much that I decided that I would start a school of my own, designed to instill drive in students. I wanted them to have passion about life and to create futures full of purpose and fun. Since I loved the arts and knew of their potential to get kids moving in the right direction, I created Renaissance Academy, a school for the arts, in 2003. In the beginning, we had even more problems with drive than more established schools. Students were coming to our school because of these issues, so almost all of them lacked drive. We learned so much in the first couple of years and applied it to our curriculum, instruction, and support for parents. This book is intended to help you put those principles into practice and turn your kids into the movers and shakers of the future.

Creating Drive: Maria's Story

Remember Maria from the beginning of this chapter? Maria enrolled in our school when she was in sixth grade. She was very shy and didn't seem to want to do much of anything. Before coming to us, she could barely read and had very little interest in academics, friends, or other activities.

Maria's mom, Kim, was becoming more and more concerned. She knew Maria was capable of so much. When Maria was younger, Kim knew how important it was to get her child active in things and had Maria involved in just about everything. From the time Maria was a toddler, she had been taking dance lessons and horseback-riding lessons, playing soccer, going on playdates, and doing lots of other fun activities. That's why it seemed so strange to Kim that Maria no longer took much of an interest in anything.

Kim was determined to take action and help Maria gain the skills she needed to become a successful adult. Kim decided to get Maria away from her old friends, who seemed to have the same disinterest in life. Kim enrolled her in our school because of its emphasis on the arts. She remembered how Maria's face lit up when she was a little girl and put on a tutu and thought if Maria could somehow find that spark, she might once again develop the drive she so desperately needed to succeed.

Maria rebelled. She couldn't believe her mom would just yank her away from her friends at school. She shut down even more, and it was a battle to get her to school each day.

At Renaissance Academy, Maria had to take ballet. She hated the dance teacher and thought her lessons were boring, hard, and pointless. One day, the teacher made Maria perform a step over and over again in front of all the other kids. Maria was mortified. She went home and cried to her mom, vowing never to come back again. (Actually, Maria constantly snuck into the bathroom to call her mom on her cell phone to complain; Kim received two or three calls a day from her daughter.)

At this point, Kim feared she had made a terrible mistake. Now her child was embarrassed on top of everything else. Thinking it might be best if Maria switched to a different class, Kim decided to visit the school with Maria to talk to the dance teacher and the principal.

In the meeting, the teacher explained that she believed Maria had a lot of talent and that she was pushing her because she knew Maria could be really good. Meanwhile, the principal said that

Maria would have to stay in the class until the end of the semester. Maria was not sure what to make of all this. In the past when her mom complained, the school gave in and promised the teachers wouldn't be so mean or just moved her to another teacher. But somehow this was different. The dance teacher seemed to want to make Maria do things, seemed to think she was capable. Maria and her mom agreed she would stay in school even if it meant staying in the dance class. Soon it was the end of the semester, and the dance class was performing in a school production. Maria was not the best kid on the stage, but she was good—she had learned everything and performed her steps properly. She made a couple of mistakes, but she covered them well, so nobody in the audience could tell. She remembered to keep her head up and hold her hands in the right position. She felt so accomplished! The following semester, Maria decided to stay in the school—and the dance class.

Time went by and Maria found success in other areas as well. She began to talk about going to college and getting a part-time job. Suddenly, her mom couldn't hold her back. Maria wanted to try new things and was eager to visit new places. She was no longer the shy, fearful girl she once was. She learned to delay gratification, to become less dependent on her mom, and to be rewarded for only true achievement. Maria had developed drive and was using it to live her life to the fullest.

Maria is one of countless students who came to Renaissance Academy with no direction, no motivation, and no will to succeed. Thanks to our wonderful faculty, carefully coordinated curriculum, and planned activities and strategies, we are developing drive in all our students. This book will show you the strategies that you can use at home to develop kids who are driven to lead happy, healthy lives.

Simply put, drive is the need or desire to accomplish. People with high levels of drive will manage risks and overcome obstacles in pursuit of a particular goal. They will understand what is most important in their life in a given timeframe and focus on that, moving forward with a singular purpose and laserlike focus. Drive is what separates high achievers from low achievers.

Does your child have the drive needed for life? Read on, and learn how to create drive in your child.

The Driving Test

How Motivated Is Your Child?

Mark, age sixteen, sometimes shows up for school on time, and sometimes doesn't. His mother is frustrated. "I try as hard as I can to get him up for school each morning," she says, to no avail. She can't figure out what the problem is. "It is almost as if he is an infant again, unable to distinguish between day and night! He will go on the computer or watch TV or talk on the phone until two or three in the morning, sometimes falling asleep on the couch. When it is time to get up for school, he is dead to the world without any sense of urgency to get up and go to school."

Mark's mom begs, pleads, cajoles, threatens, and once even threw a little water on him to get him up for school. Eventually, Mark will get up, but he is usually late. Once he finally gets to school, he doesn't really engage. Though he used to be a good student, he is now very tired and lethargic, and he can't seem to get interested in very much. His mom tries to get him to understand the importance of school and offers him rewards for good grades.

She thinks she has the ultimate carrot: a driver's license. She has told Mark time and again that he will not be able to get his license unless his grades improve. Did this work? "I couldn't believe it," his mother reports. "Now Mark doesn't seem to care about a driver's license or anything else! He is perfectly content to just sit at home and play video games." Mark's behavior is strongly similar to a teen who smokes pot and becomes apathetic about life in general. Although Mark's mom doesn't believe he is smoking pot, she has tested him for drugs a couple of times just to be sure. Mark isn't using drugs; he simply doesn't care about anything.

Every day with Mark is a struggle. Him mom feels as if she is carrying her son's responsibilities and doing too much for him because he cannot seem to get himself moving. She worries that he will not finish high school and will not have the desire to leave home when he is older.

Clearly, Mark suffers from a lack of drive. What caused the demise of Mark's inner motivation? He has grown up in a luxurious world where everything is programmed for him, things are very safe, he has been rewarded for each successful task, and things are given to him as soon as he requests them. From the time he was a very young child, his parents provided for his every desire, and now he really doesn't desire anything.

Drive Versus Desire

Drive is often confused with desire. Desire just means that you want something. Drive is the willingness to do what it takes to get it. It is not enough to want something, and many parents too quickly give in when their children express certain desires. Giving children whatever they want when they want it actually diminishes drive. Over time, if a child is always given what he wants without earning it, he will never experience the deep yearning that will motivate him to achieve.

For example, some young children, particularly girls, express a desire to have a horse. They whine and carry on, sometimes for years, to convince their parents to buy the horse. If this goes on long enough, a parent might believe that this expressed desire, combined with relentless badgering, equals drive. However, that is not true. A child who desires a horse may talk about horses constantly, read stories about horses, and plead for a horse. A child who is driven to get a horse will also begin saving money, offer to work at a local barn in exchange for riding privileges, sign up for lessons at a local stable, and engage in other meaningful activities that will result in time around or on horses. She will do whatever she has to do to be close to these wonderful creatures. She will forgo other things in her life to save money and find the time necessary to achieve this goal.

Like Mark, many young people are obsessed with video games. They eat, sleep, and breathe their favorite game, forgoing all else. Although some parents may be concerned about such behavior, they are often happy to see their child passionate about something. They may believe that this passion will one day translate into a career for their child, who may state that he wants to be a game designer. Is this drive? Usually not. Although there are a few people who will turn this obsession into a career, it is not normally the case. Most people who get obsessed in this way will avoid all other priorities for the video game, which can actually turn into a type of addiction. It is critical to differentiate between your children's desire and drive so you can help them develop lifelong passions.

An extreme example of parents who confuse desire with drive can be found on a recent television reality series that chronicled the lives of families who were helping their children become professional actors. One of the stories centered on a single mom who moved with her daughters to Los Angeles. The mother sacrificed her marriage, her career, her home, and her life in Nevada to help her older daughter pursue the dream of becoming an actor. Certainly,

The Difference Between Desire and Drive	
Desire	*Drive*
A young girl constantly pesters her parents to buy her a horse.	A young girl rides her bike to the stable so she can clean stalls in hopes of being able to ride a horse.
A young boy plays video games constantly and says he wants to be a game designer.	A young boy creates his own computer games, reads about game design, and talks to others who are in the profession.

there was no question about the mom's drive to help her daughter reach this goal.

However, in episode after episode, viewers watched the daughter fail to prepare for auditions, complain about difficult conditions, and choose to play instead of working at classes and other activities that would improve her chances of success. In one episode, the mother cried because she knew how much her daughter wanted to act, and she was running out of money. She felt that she was letting her daughter down because they had to move back to Nevada. The daughter blamed her mother for her own lack of success and decided to move into a friend's house to continue pursuing her dream. The mother allowed her to do so and felt like a failure because her daughter had not yet succeeded.

What Does Drive Look Like?

At what age would you like your child to move out of your house? Twenty? Thirty? Forty? If you would like your child to get beyond the walls of your house, you must assist him in developing drive. People with drive have many advantages over those without it:

A person with drive finishes things. Drive provides you the follow-through to get things done. A person with drive understands how important it is to finish things and honor his responsibilities. A driven person focuses on the goal and is always working to move closer toward it.

A person with drive has the determination to have healthy lifelong relationships. A balanced person who has drive will want to make all the parts of his life work well together. Driven people who have life partners approach the maintenance of their relationships with as much gusto as they do other things that are important to them. This focus and work make relationships successful.

A person with drive finds fulfillment in work. A driven person finds joy in work because he has a sense of purpose. Many highly driven people have difficulty understanding the concept of retirement, opting to focus on different priorities instead of heading for the golf course. Work should be exciting enough to make you want to get up in the morning to get things done. Driven people understand this concept and live it every day.

A person with drive usually earns more money. If you have drive, you will generally want more out of life and understand the hard work that is required to get these things. Even a person who is motivated by very altruistic goals understands the importance of money in reaching those goals. Develop drive, and the money will follow.

A person with drive can deal with uncertainty and change. Driven people understand the normal ups and downs of life. They are able to work through difficulties and crises because they understand that things will get better. Work, persistence, and goal orientation make this possible.

A person with drive leads an interesting life. A person with drive is continually trying new things and seeking new adventures. A person with drive enjoys making things happen and bringing others along for the ride. A life with drive is rich and full and wonderful!

How much drive does your child currently have? Take one of the tests that follow to find out. (A rating scale to interpret your answers appears on page 32.)

Drive Questionnaire for Middle and High School Students

1. Does your child get up for school on time without much prompting?
2. Can your child talk about at least three interests other than hanging out, chatting online, talking on the phone, surfing the Net, playing video games, or going to the mall?
3. Does your child complete all of his or her schoolwork without much prompting?
4. Is your child able to talk about the kind of future he or she dreams about?
5. Does your child save money for things he or she wants?
6. Does your child complete activities such as a sports season or a role in a play?
7. Is your child involved in extracurricular activities?
8. Is your child a good traveler?
9. Do your child's stated desires and behaviors match? (Example: The child says that she wants to make the cheerleading squad, and she practices endlessly before the tryouts.)
10. Does your child attend school at least 95 percent of the time?

11. Does your child enjoy talking to you about his or her day?

12. Does your child like spending time with you and talking with you?

13. Is your child looking forward to driving a car as soon as possible?

14. Does your child regularly engage in physical activities such as bike riding, tree climbing, and walking?

15. Does your child have a good balance of structured activities and downtime?

16. Does your child seek opportunities to travel, participate in competitions or festivals, or attend special events?

17. Does your child have a true passion about something?

18. Does your child regularly set goals that lead him or her toward a purpose in life?

19. Does your child work at a job or help neighbors to earn money?

↑ Drive Questionnaire for Full-Time College Students

1. Is your child enrolled in at least fifteen credits each semester?
2. Does your child demonstrate interest in some classes?
3. Does your child talk with you about college?
4. Does your child socialize with other students at college?
5. Does your child live on campus or have a desire to move away from home sometime within the next year?
6. Does your child go on road trips or attend concerts or other special events with friends?
7. Can your child talk about at least three interests other than hanging out, chatting online, talking on the phone, surfing the Net, playing video games, or going to the mall?
8. Does your child complete school assignments on time?
9. Is your child a good traveler?
10. Do your child's stated desires and behaviors match? (Example: The child says that she wants to go on a vacation and works tirelessly to earn the money to go.)
11. Does your child attend school at least 95 percent of the time?
12. Does your child enjoy talking to you about his or her day?
13. Does your child like spending time and talking with you?
14. Does your child have a driver's license?
15. Does your child regularly engage in physical activities?
16. Does your child have a good balance of structured activities and downtime?
17. Does your child avoid the common college traps of too much alcohol and partying?
18. Does your child have a true passion about something?
19. Does your child regularly set goals that lead him or her toward a purpose in life?

Drive Questionnaire for Young Adults Not Enrolled Full-Time in School

1. Does your child work (for money or on a volunteer basis)?

2. Does your child engage in activities that result in learning and growing?

3. Is your child engaged in organized activities (work, classes, etc.) at least thirty hours a week?

4. Does your child socialize with peers?

5. Does your child have a desire to move away from home sometime within the next year?

6. Does your child go on road trips or attend concerts or other special events with friends?

7. Can your child talk about at least three interests other than hanging out, chatting online, talking on the phone, surfing the Net, playing video games, or going to the mall?

8. Does your child meet his or her obligations and responsibilities?

9. Is your child a good traveler?

10. Do your child's stated desires and behaviors match? (Example: The child says that she wants to go to college and is actively researching options.)

11. Does your child regularly attend (at least 95 percent of the time) all scheduled work and activities?

12. Does your child enjoy talking to you about his or her day?

13. Does your child like spending time with you and talking with you?

14. Does your child have a driver's license?

15. Does your child regularly engage in physical activities?

16. Does your child have a good balance of structured activities and downtime?

(continued)

17. Does your child avoid the common traps of too much alcohol and partying?

18. Does your child have a true passion about something?

19. Does your child regularly set goals that lead him or her toward a purpose in life?

Drive Questionnaire Rating Scale

To how many of the questions on a single questionnaire did you answer yes?

0–4 Your child is in great need of improving drive.

5–9 Your child has some short-term motivation but needs assistance in developing true drive.

10–14 Your child has some drive but could use more direction.

15–19 Your child is on the right track and on the road to success.

If you scored your child's drive from 0 to 9, he is likely to grow up and continue to inhabit your home, may or may not pay rent, and may or may not do his fair share around the house. If, on the other hand, you would like to get your child out of your house and into a life of his own, read on and help him drive toward a great future.

If you scored your child's drive from 10 to 14, you are on the right track. However, you need to employ some simple techniques included in this book to keep nudging him past any fear and on to great things.

If you scored your child's drive from 15 to 19, congratulations! You have done a good job of instilling drive in your child. Keep doing what has worked for you, and enjoy getting to know your child as an adult. Give this book to a friend!

Now that you understand your child's drive, it is time to learn about how your parenting style has impacted his drive. In the next chapter, I will help you understand how to parent to increase drive in your teen or young adult. Once you understand yourself as a parent, you will be ready to implement the first drive strategy. As a "pathfinder parent," you will learn to obtain critical information about your child and use that information to propel you both forward.

1. Be a Pathfinder

Gather the Info That Really Makes a Difference

Lisa was so excited to begin kindergarten! She was five years old and had a new dress for the occasion. She was a little nervous and held tightly to her mom's hand as they entered the classroom—but the teacher was so nice and friendly. The teacher told Lisa to put her backpack on the shelf with her name on it and sit at the desk with her name on it. Lisa had just a little tear in her eye as she said good-bye to her mom and took her seat. She knew everything would be OK and was eager to get started.

But Elaine, Lisa's mom, was worried. She knew that Lisa would not be able to function on her own. Lisa had never been in school before; everything would be so strange. So Elaine stood in the hall by the classroom door and watched, ready to rush in if Lisa needed her. Ten minutes later, when the principal came down the hall and told her it was OK to go, Elaine just could not leave. She said, "I am not going. I don't think she is ready to leave me yet." The principal tried to reassure her but was unsuccessful. Elaine stayed at school for the entire day. At lunch Elaine popped in to see Lisa, who cried as soon as she saw her mom. For Elaine that was more evidence that Lisa was not ready to leave her. When Lisa went to recess, her mom stood by the tree next to the kickball field, certain that Lisa would not know what to do or would fall down. Elaine stood guard the entire time, even when the teacher led Lisa away from her to participate in the game.

Over the years, Lisa progressed through school. Although Elaine no longer stood guard at recess, she was there every step of the way. She made sure that Lisa's teachers understood when there was a good reason for Lisa to have incomplete homework. She intervened when Lisa had arguments with friends and made sure that Lisa's teachers always knew if Lisa needed something. Elaine was always there to bring forgotten items to school and to take Lisa home at the first sign of discomfort. Lisa was Elaine's world, and Elaine wanted everything to be perfect for her daughter all the time.

Fast-forward several more years, and things hadn't changed. Lisa went to college, and Elaine was there, as she'd always been. Elaine moved Lisa into the dorm and talked with her adviser to make sure she was taking the right classes. Elaine also made a color-coded schedule for Lisa so she could get to all her classes. She called Lisa on the phone every day to wake her up for classes, usually calling at least twice to ensure Lisa was up. Whenever there was a question about an assignment or grade, Elaine dutifully e-mailed the professor to get clarification. Elaine edited all of Lisa's papers and even came every other weekend to clean her dorm room and to do her laundry. Thank goodness for Elaine; Lisa would never have been able to manage in college without her!

Helicopter Parents

Of course, it's important to be involved in your child's life and provide guidance. But Elaine is more than involved; she is a helicopter parent. She hovers over her daughter to watch Lisa's every move and make sure Lisa is safe from harm. Elaine doesn't want Lisa to make any mistakes and swoops in whenever there is danger. If Lisa does have any problem, Elaine is there to pull her up and fly her away before things get too stressful.

Many parents fall into the trap of hovering over their children. They are always there, always intervening, always directing, always rescuing. These helicopter parents, while well intentioned, don't allow their children to experience the natural process of separating from them and developing into independent adults.

Hot Air Balloon Parents

Joe was a high school student whose parents were nothing like Lisa's mom. Theresa and Frank knew they needed to give Joe room to grow and make his own mistakes. Frank believed that Joe would probably make some of the same mistakes that he did and was not surprised to learn that Joe had smoked pot a few times with friends. However, when Frank found out, he didn't want to confront Joe; he believed that it was perfectly normal for a teenager to dabble in relatively harmless drugs. As Frank said, "The more a parent pushes, the more likely he will push his child away, right?" Frank wanted to remain good friends with his son and believed that he shouldn't demand information or ask Joe to comply with unnecessary rules. So he and Theresa "just kind of let Joe do his own thing."

When Joe started college a few months ago, Theresa and Frank hoped things would go OK. Overall, Joe is a pretty good kid, but Frank knew Joe would probably continue to make mistakes. As the semester came to a close, Frank hoped that his son had been going to classes and doing his work. He hoped that Joe was not partying too much and that he was choosing good friends.

When Joe came home for winter break, he told his dad that he did not want to return for the spring term. He said that college was not for him and that he just wanted to move back home and work for a while. Frank thought this would be OK and did not want to butt into Joe's life. Finally, Joe admitted to his dad that he had failed most of his classes because he often didn't show up. It turns out that Joe had been partying constantly and did not focus on his studies at all.

Frank is a hot air balloon parent. He lets his son do most of the steering, kind of like the wind carrying a hot air balloon. A hot air balloon parent can adjust things a little bit but does not have the power to really make his child do the right things.

Hot air balloon parents kind of go along for the ride. They believe that their children will make the same mistakes they did, or worse, and that there is really not much they can do to impact their children's decisions. This type of parenting can have disastrous results.

Pathfinder Parents

Instead of acting like a helicopter or hot air balloon, parents need to have a range of approaches to help their child move toward adulthood. Consider the pathfinder in the military. This critical position involves going ahead of the troops to gain vital information so they can move forward. The pathfinder is always on the lookout for weather patterns, enemy movements, and environmental hazards. This information is then funneled to the rest of the unit so that important decisions can be made. Likewise, pathfinder parents must investigate to learn about anything that may impact their child on the uncharted path.

A good parent will scout the path ahead of her child to help that child make good decisions. She will identify hidden dangers (e.g., unmotivated friends, a lack of education, poor health, toxic relationships); potential threats (e.g., alcohol, drugs, dangerous hobbies); and places out of harm's way (e.g., good peer groups, schools, jobs, opportunities). The job of a pathfinder parent is to know what may happen next and to deliver that information to her child in a manner that is helpful and well received by the child. Only then will her findings be truly useful. The key is that the child perceives that the parent is actually on his side. Children tend to perceive the parent as the enemy, instead of the advance team that they need to keep away from the land mines and ditches along the road to adulthood. A pathfinder parent keeps her child on the right path to becoming a happy, successful adult.

Lorraine and Chris have a beautiful daughter named Chelsea who is a high school freshman. Like most parents, they worry all the time. They want to protect Chelsea from harm but also know they must allow her to gain independence and confidence. Last year they became very concerned about Chelsea. She seemed withdrawn and sad. She wasn't sleeping well, and they had difficulty getting her going in the morning. They kept questioning her—talking about school, friends, and everything else they thought might be the problem—to no avail. Then they started noticing that every time they got close to her when she was on the computer, she would quickly minimize the screen. They suspected something was happening online. They tried talking to her about it, but she would not tell them anything. They tried looking at her browser history, but she was smart enough to clear that every time. The more Lorraine and Chris probed, the less Chelsea talked. Chris decided to learn more about where Chelsea was going online. He found software that would allow him to track her history without her knowledge. After just a couple of days, Chris was able to track Chelsea's activities to a social-networking site. Chris went right to her and asked her to explain. Chelsea turned red and began sobbing. She told her dad everything.

↑ What Kind of Parent Are You?

You may be a helicopter parent if:

- Your child has difficulty separating from you to go to school or out with friends.
- You bail him out whenever he gets into trouble.
- You believe he really needs you around all the time.
- You intervene with teachers every time he is concerned about something, instead of teaching him how to do it himself. (Have you ever caught yourself saying something like, "Hello, Mr. Smith. My son is in your second-period math class, and he would like to know the requirements of the class project"? Or "Hi, Mrs. Adams. My daughter doesn't understand why you put her in the group with Sarah. You know she and Sarah don't get along. She would like to be put in a different group"?)
- You manage every movement your child makes. You wake him in the mornings even though he is sixteen years old. You watch the clock so he doesn't take too long of a shower. You tell him exactly when and how to do every little thing.
- You review your child's homework and make any necessary changes. You are your child's personal secretary, providing scheduling, typing, and phone services whenever necessary.
- You do the legwork in making appointments, arranging rides, and managing every detail of your teen's life.

You may be a hot air balloon parent if:

- Your child has seemed really down lately, but you have chosen not to confront her about it because you don't want to pry.

- Your child is late to school at least twice a week, but you figure she just needs to learn to do things on her own.
- You rarely or never check to see if your child's homework is done because it's all up to her—after all, it's her assignment.
- You don't really have a close relationship with your child. She never confides in you, asks for guidance, or asks for your opinion.
- You ignore the signs that your child is smoking pot (or using other substances) because you figure all kids are bound to try it sooner or later, and mentioning it may encourage her to smoke more.

You may be a pathfinder parent if:

- You really listen to your child and ensure that the two of you spend time together.
- You know who your child's friends are.
- You know where your child is at all times.
- You help your child solve his own problems with minimal intervention.
- When your child makes a mistake, you allow him to suffer the consequences.
- You provide appropriate punishments and follow through on them.
- You step in when the consequences of a mistake could be life threatening or life altering.

Chelsea had signed up for this site, even though her parents had explicitly told her not to. She created a profile of herself, complete with a fictitious age and provocative photo. Through this site, Chelsea had entered into a cyberrelationship with someone claiming to be a seventeen-year-old young man. Chelsea had fallen for him, and he was now being nasty to her, calling her names and arguing with her online. Because Chris had the information he needed, he was able to help Chelsea. Together they shut down the site. This experience opened the door to productive conversations about relationships, cybersafety, and life in general. A helicopter parent would have intruded on Chelsea to the point that she would have become more secretive. A hot air balloon parent would have dismissed Chelsea's mood, attributing it to normal adolescence. Chelsea's pathfinder parents were able to get the information they needed to help their daughter avoid danger and find a safe place.

Although a child is by no means the enemy, his purposes are oftentimes in complete conflict with his parents' priorities or wishes. Pathfinders are constantly, quietly working to stay one step ahead of their child. The parent who pulls this off is admired, even revered, by his child for his uncanny ability to predict the future and see things the child thought had been so skillfully hidden from view. A child must believe, when faced with a questionable circumstance, that he will be found out, that his parents have eyes on the backs of their heads, and that they carry a crystal ball that predicts his actions.

The truth is that most children, teens, and even young adults are very predictable in their daily behavior. They throw us occasional curveballs when selecting a career, choosing a mate, and making other life-changing decisions. However, their daily comings and goings happen almost like clockwork. We can unwittingly set the stage for their undesirable behavior. For example, if we make excuses for our kids when they fail to complete a homework assignment, they will frequently "forget" to do homework assignments. If they hang out with certain friends who bring out the worst in them, they will be determined to befriend those kids and will misbehave as a result. The key to keeping kids on the right track so they are driven to success is paying attention to what they are doing, anticipating the dangers and threats that may come along. You can allow them enough freedom to make the mistakes that will help them learn and grow while intervening when their errors will put them in true danger. A pathfinder parent stealthily garners the data necessary to continually analyze dangers and help his child navigate safely into adulthood.

Stealth Reconnaissance

When Lisa was a teenager, Elaine—a helicopter mom—always made sure she got all the information she needed to impact her daughter's life. She read Lisa's diary and regularly rummaged through Lisa's drawers, closet, and personal belongings. She listened in on telephone conversations, read Lisa's e-mails, and eavesdropped when Lisa had friends over. Every time there was anything that raised a concern, Elaine confronted Lisa about it. Lisa knew her mom was always looking over her shoulder and intruding, so she developed ingenious ways to hide things. Instead of encouraging Lisa to behave better, Elaine was actually teaching her to be secretive and sneaky.

Children naturally desire to separate from their parents beginning at about age ten or eleven. By the time they are teens, they believe that friendships are all important and will fight to the death to preserve them. If a parent is too intrusive, the child will simply retreat more and become very adept at covering her tracks. Elaine believes that she knows everything about her daughter. However, she only knows what Lisa will allow her to know. Lisa doesn't trust her mom because she thinks her mom is always interfering. This actually decreases the amount of knowledge Elaine can gain from Lisa, and it forces Lisa to lie and hide things.

How to Be an Involved Parent without Hovering

So what is a parent to do? How do you find out the important aspects of your children's life while respecting their privacy and not being overly intrusive? Your children should always believe that you somehow could find out everything. For example, even if they lie to you about where they are going, you could always call up a friend's mom and learn the truth. Only then will a teen or young adult stop and think before doing things that you may not approve of.

Know Where Your Child Is at All Times

Every time your child goes out unsupervised, get a detailed itinerary from her. Ask her where she is going and with whom. Ask her who is driving, when she expects to arrive, and what time she'll be home. If plans change, let her know that you expect her to call you before proceeding to the next location.

If you suspect she is not being truthful about her whereabouts, occasionally show up at one of the locations unannounced. You can make up a reason to allow her to save face with her friends, saying, "Oh, I was just on my way to pick up the dry cleaning and noticed Mrs. Smith's car; I thought I would stop by and see if you needed any more money" or "I couldn't reach your cell phone, so I wanted to be sure you are OK. Is your battery dead?" If she is not where she is supposed to be, track her down and take her home promptly.

Be Clear That Drug and Alcohol Use Is Not Acceptable

If you suspect your child is smoking, drinking, or using any type of substance, you absolutely should search his room and belongings. If

---

↑ Signs That Your Child May Be
Smoking Cigarettes

If you suspect that your child may smoke, ask yourself these questions:

- Have you smelled smoke on her clothing or hair?

- Have you seen matches in her bedroom or a lighter in her backpack?

- Has she started making excuses to go outside?

- Has she been leaving the windows in her bedroom open for no reason?

- Are there burn holes in her clothing?

- Has she started using mouthwash, breath mints, or gum?

- Does she have friends who smoke?

Source: Philip Morris Youth Smoking Prevention Web Site (www.pmusa.com)

---

you don't find anything, he should never know that you searched. This is critical. If he knows you are snooping, he will just get better at hiding it.

If you do find evidence that your child is using an illegal substance, try confronting him with the truth without revealing the search. Focus on the behavior that led you to suspect drug or alcohol abuse in the first place. For example, if your child was slurring his words and stumbling but denied drinking and you found evidence otherwise, talk about what could cause slurred speech and stumbling. If he still denies it, tell him that you are very concerned and think you might need to get him to the doctor because these are warning signs of strokes and other neurological disorders. Ask him what he thinks could possibly cause this behavior. Then tell

---

↑ Signs That Your Child May Be Using
Drugs or Alcohol

If you suspect that your child may use drugs or alcohol, ask
yourself these questions:

- Has your child had a recent change in his group of
  friends?
- Does he lie about his whereabouts?
- Has he had a dramatic personality or mood change?
- Does he frequently make excuses for not being able to
  attend family events or outings?
- Does he use incense, room spray, or perfumes (which
  hide smoke or chemical odors)?
- Does he use secretive or coded language with friends?
- Has he been taking money without explaining how he's
  spending it?

---

him that you know what he is doing. If he still denies it, say, "So if
we were to go together right now into your room, we would not
find anything that shouldn't be there, right? Because I really hope I
am wrong about this." If he still denies it, go together to his room,
and search the places where you know you will find something.

By focusing on the behavior that led you to the suspicion,
your child will learn that you care enough to notice him and what
he is doing. Be prepared, however, for him to complain that you
have violated his privacy, which always comes with a room search.
If he does complain, stress that his room is in *your* house. You
need to walk the fine line of allowing your child to become his

- Has your child been in trouble—with family, at work or school, or with the police—because of drinking or drug use?

- Have you found evidence of drug paraphernalia, such as pipes or rolling papers?

- Have you found inhaling products—such as hairspray, nail polish, and correction fluid—or rags and paper bags (which are sometimes used as inhalant accessories)?

- Have you found bottles of eye drops (which may be used to mask bloodshot eyes or dilated pupils)?

- Has your child come home after school or after being out with the smell of mouthwash or breath mints (which are used to cover up the smell of alcohol)?

- Have you been missing any prescription drugs or cold medicines?

Source: Partnership for a Drug-Free America Web Site (www.drugfree.org)

own person, with his own space, while maintaining the right to make the rules.

What's next for the parent who discovers that her child is abusing a substance—whether it's tobacco, alcohol, prescription drugs, illegal drugs, inhalants, or over-the-counter medications? You need to take swift, aggressive action on the issue. After confronting your child with what you know, focus on the following:

- *Reduce or eliminate your child's access to the substance.* You will need to take extreme measures to remove anything from your home that will tempt your child. This may include all aerosol cans if your child is abusing inhalants. It may mean *you* will need to stop smoking if your child is smoking. It may mean that *you* forgo alcohol if your child is abusing that. If there are substances you must keep in the home that may be a temptation, purchase a small safe in which to keep them and put it in your bedroom closet. However, be forewarned: if you regularly smoke, drink, or use drugs and you don't quit, chances are your child will continue the same behavior. If you don't want your child following the same path, what better motivation will you ever have to quit?

- *Reduce your child's access to friends who are abusing the substance.* Whenever possible, do not allow your child to be with this peer group.
- *Frequently search your child's room, backpack, and other belongings.* Be stealthy. Be unpredictable.
- *Get help from professionals.* Determine what type of counseling and rehab your child needs, and secure it immediately. Require your child to participate.

Put the Computer in a "Public" Location at Home

Don't allow your child to have a computer in her bedroom. Instead, restrict your child's online activities to a computer that is centrally located in the house, like in the kitchen or family room. Pick the place with the most traffic. Watch for lots of clicking when you walk by. If you see your child quickly closing windows or changing Web sites as you get closer, she is probably hiding something. If you are worried about what she is doing, instruct her to get up, and use the back button or history tab to see where she has been.

Also be sure you know which social-networking sites—MySpace, Facebook, or others—your child frequents. You might want to help her create her profile. Talk about the types of photos that are OK to post and the types that are not. When she is not around, see whether you can find her by searching her name or nicknames. You may stumble on another profile she has created without your input. Confront her about this, and let her know how easy it was to find her so that she will understand how easy it is for a predator. Tell her that you are concerned about her safety, and help her understand what reasonable boundaries need to be in place so that she can protect herself.

No matter how hard you try, you will not be able to keep your child away from the Internet. Kids often believe that Internet predators will never find them or harm them. It is important that you talk to your child about friends online. Go through her lists of friends from a social-networking site. Have her tell you who each person is and how she knows him or her. If her only contact with a person is online, help her understand how easy it is to be deceived online. With her help, create a fictitious profile on the site. Show her that any adult can pose as a teen and lure kids into conversations. Talk about what could happen if this so-called friend manages to lure her to a physical location. Be sure she understands that this could happen to her while teaching her how to protect herself.

Know Your Child's School
Become friends with teachers, administrators, and counselors. You can volunteer with teachers and coaches who take an interest in your child. Find out what your child is really like in school: learn what social group she is a part of and how she behaves in different groups. Develop a network of adults who can alert you when something is wrong.

Volunteer to Chaperone Field Trips or Social Outings
Enjoy being around your child and her friends. Listen to what they chat about—they will reveal most of themselves when they don't think you are noticing. As you walk through the destination, pay

attention to how your child's group reacts to other students. Pay attention to their conversations and keep listening.

Make Your House the Hangout

Buy pizza and have the kids sit around the kitchen table. As they are eating, busy yourself doing chores in the kitchen. They *will* talk. Listen, listen, listen.

Ask Your Child about Her Friends

When you are alone with your daughter, ask her about her friends and what is going on in their lives. (For more on this, see chapter 10.) Use information you have obtained through conversations with her friends or their parents to steer the conversation. At this point, you need to be friendly enough to gain more information and to offer sage advice. For example, if she tells you about a friend who is doing questionable things—like cheating on tests, talking back to adults, or smoking—ask her what she thinks about that. Try using questioning techniques rather than lecturing. What does she think she might do in that situation? Ask her if she is concerned about hanging out with this person.

The Dos and Don'ts of Conducting Reconnaissance on a College Student

Although a college-age student is legally an adult, he still depends on you financially and is likely not ready to assume all the responsibilities of adulthood. This is a time to increase his independence while still ensuring his safety and well-being. A parent must gradually allow a child in college to take more and more control over his life while helping protect him from the types of errors that can cause significant harm—such as running up major credit card debt. Excellent reconnaissance that is not overly intrusive is the key to learning what you need to do to successfully guide your college student in a positive way.

Do

- Set up a joint checking account the first year your child is away from you. Be sure it is at a bank that has branches in your hometown and is convenient to where your child is living. Set up online banking, and check on his activities frequently.
- Sit down with your child, and set up his college's online services so that you have access to and can check on schedules, grades, and so on.
- Have a meeting with your child's counselor and your child to review degree requirements, course loads, and so forth.
- Help your child just before and just after the first semester begins to locate classrooms, to determine his transportation needs, and to determine how much time he will need to get to class on time.
- Set up a meal plan that will ensure your child will not go hungry, even if he spends all his money on other things.
- Arrange for any necessary public transportation at the beginning of the semester so that your child can get to class, even if he spends all his money on other things.
- Discuss your child's spending habits with him to help him make good financial decisions.
- Instruct your child to shred every credit card offer that he receives. Instruct him not to apply for credit to get discounts or freebies.
- Set up a family plan for your child's cell phone that provides plenty of minutes so that he can call home whenever necessary.
- Have a continual dialogue about classes, finances, health, and nutrition.

- Monitor use of the meal plan if that is available to you. If you cannot access it online, you can probably call the bursar's office and ask for a printout of activity.
- Check your child's credit report, and discuss it with him at least once a year.

Don't
- Contact your child's instructors, professors, or counselors directly once he starts college.
- Provide daily wake-up calls for your child.
- Give your child money every time he asks for it.
- Check on his cell phone usage and track calls.
- Bail him out by giving him more of things he has failed to use or budget properly.
- Allow him to come home so often that he doesn't take part in university life.

Intervention Levels

The process of reconnaissance provides parents with vital information. Once that information is obtained, it is critical to understand the type of intervention that will be most effective. A pathfinder parent gets the information early and often to understand the mistakes that her child is about to make. She then assesses the risk and determines what level of intervention is necessary:

- No intervention is required if the consequence will cause a minor inconvenience, like the loss of a little of your child's money or a disappointment. Leave it alone, and let natural consequences take hold.
- Intervention is required if the consequence will cause a major inconvenience, negatively affect other people, cost your child a lot of money, or create a devastating disappointment. Coach,

↑ Serenity Prayer for Parents

God, grant me the serenity to accept the mistakes my child
must make in order to learn, the courage to step in when
the consequences are too great, and the wisdom to know the
difference.

question, and advise—but then allow the child to make the
decision and suffer the consequences. Be sure your child
understands that you will not bail him out if things go awry.

- Aggressive intervention is required if the consequence will be
  life altering, causing the loss of future opportunities necessary
  for success (such as continuation in school, good health, etc.).
  Step in immediately and take aggressive action to intervene.

Reconnecting with Your Child

The most important part of being a parent is developing a relationship with your kids that allows you to stay connected with them
throughout their lives. Even if you feel as if you have lost that connection, or didn't have it in the first place, it is never too late to get
connected. All you have to do is find some common ground.
Pathfinder parents are continually looking for connections and creating ones that allow them into their kids' lives.

Howard Walker thought that he was missing out on his three
daughters' fleeting teen years. He worked long hours during the
week and frequently had to travel out of town. His girls were growing up too quickly, and he felt as if he didn't even know them. On
weekends they were off doing things with their friends and didn't

really have time for their old dad. During the winter months, they spent nearly every Saturday skiing in the mountains, which was several hours away. On the one day a week that he could spend with them, they would be gone for over twelve hours!

But Howard Walker had a plan. He decided to secretly take skiing lessons so he could join his girls on the slopes. One Saturday he volunteered to chauffeur them to the mountains and drove the three hours to the snow. When they arrived, the girls and their friends got out of the car and took their skis off the roof rack. Howard got out of the car and headed to the large trunk. When they weren't looking, he took out *his* new skis, strapped them on his feet, and skied right past his three girls! Everyone was stunned. When did their father learn to ski? He was actually pretty good at it! From that point on, Howard was the designated driver to the mountains. He spent nearly every Saturday in the car—six hours!—with his girls and their friends and went down the slopes with them. He learned about school, friends, boyfriends (when they thought he wasn't listening), fears, accomplishments, and everything else parents should know about their kids. He listened a lot but never offered much advice. He just channeled the information to his wife, who used it when she had her many heart-to-heart conversations with their daughters.

And this is a true story—Howard Walker is my dad. Although he no longer skis, he still enjoys a close relationship with my sisters and me. He wasn't interested in skiing initially, although he did grow to love it. He was looking for a way to connect with his children and to gain important information that he needed to parent.

What have you done with your kids lately? A great way to stay involved in your kids' lives is to go where they are. What do they like to do? What can you do to join in the fun? It doesn't have to be as extreme as taking up a brand-new sport. It can be as simple as going for walks, going to the beach, taking trips to the mall, or playing cards or video games. The key is to go into their territory—like any good pathfinder.

Like most things in life, good parenting involves finding a good balance. You don't want to hover. You don't want to just go where the wind takes you. You want to find a path and follow it. Driven kids have parents who understand when to let them go and when to step in and help. Use excellent reconnaissance to determine the reality of your child's life. Use that information to help your child move toward a positive future.

In the next chapter, you will learn about risk taking. Every good pathfinder understands how to assess risks. Keep reading to learn how to encourage your child to take the risks that will allow him or her to gain the confidence and competence for a successful life.

2. Increase Risk
Take Away the Plastic Bubble

I grew up in a sprawling suburb in New Jersey in a very typical new development where all the streets were named after colleges. When I was four, I couldn't wait to learn to ride a two-wheeled bike so that I could keep up with my big sisters. They got to go tooling all around the neighborhood with the rest of the kids. As a matter of fact, I couldn't wait to do most things and never wanted to be left out or left behind, although I was always the smallest one (and even today measure only a shade over five feet tall).

I kept asking for a bicycle. It was just a month or so before my fifth birthday, so I kept pestering, believing that I could certainly wear my parents down before the big day. I was extremely tiny at this point and not particularly coordinated or physically skilled for my age. About a week before my birthday, my mom said that if I could learn to ride a bike—no training wheels—before my birthday, she would buy me one. I think she made that statement to make me stop pestering, never thinking for a moment that I could actually master this skill in time for my birthday.

My cousin let me use his old bike to practice. Our driveway curved up a slight hill, so I would start at the top and sort of leap onto the red seat and roll down the hill into the street. I didn't want any help. Over and over again, I jumped onto the red seat, rolled down the hill, and fell as the bike reached the street. This went on for several days. I was bruised and scraped from head to toe, but luckily, I'd learned to steer the bike toward the grass so that there was a little more cushion for each impact with the ground. This was 1967, so we didn't have bicycle helmets or padding of any kind. When you fell, you got hurt.

A few days into the ordeal, I somehow started to feel how the bike could be balanced beneath me. I felt in control for a brief moment before finding that now familiar spot on the grass where I would inevitably fall. This was encouraging, so I tried it yet again. This time I fell a little bit farther toward the road, so I did it again. Within a few more attempts, I learned to ride a bike. I never used training wheels or had anyone holding on to the seat and running behind me. My mom stood back and watched as I fell and got up, only to fall again, for what must have been dozens of times over many days in my driveway. Looking back on it, I can't believe she was able to do that. As my children were growing up, it was very difficult to allow them the bumps and bruises of life that I knew they needed to experience.

By the time I was really riding, it was just one day before my fifth birthday. Somehow my parents got to the store and bought the exact bike I wanted in time for the big day. It was a purple Schwinn, like the one both my sisters had, of course. From that point on, I rode everywhere with them, always peddling a little bit harder to keep up with all the kids who were so much bigger than I was.

The Plastic Bubble

Have you ever watched a coming-of-age movie like *Stand by Me*, *Now and Then*, or *The Sandlot*? These movies include groups of children playing and having adventures together. The characters are presented with great challenges and work together to resolve the matter at hand. They are without adult supervision for much of the time. They don't have cell phones or any contact with adults who can help, so they must rely on themselves and their own instincts to solve problems. These children take great risks as they navigate through the dangers and end up growing tremendously through their experiences.

While problems in these movies are more extreme than most children will ever experience, they illustrate beautifully how adversity, challenge, and risk help us grow. It is no accident that these movies are usually set in the early 1980s or before. During those times, children were expected to roam free. When I was growing up in the '60s and '70s, we were *not allowed* to come into the house until dinnertime! We had to play with our friends and invent our own fun. Some of my fondest memories of my preteen and early-adolescent years involve riding bikes through our neighborhood, climbing trees, walking along creeks, and even finding dinosaur bones in the park down the street. We chased dogs, watched the neighbors who we believed were in the mob, invented stories, and imagined vivid scenarios that involved heroes and villains. Yes, there were some bumps and bruises along the way; we made some mistakes and did get into trouble occasionally. But I credit these experiences with helping me become more self-reliant and independent.

In contrast, many of my students spend their afternoons differently. Steven, age thirteen, comes home every day after school at about three thirty. He gets off the bus and uses his key to get into the house and locks the door securely behind him. The first thing he does is call his mom to let her know that he is home safe. Then he turns on the TV and either plays video games or watches cartoons while he munches on snacks until his mom gets home, at about five thirty. Steven has been engaged in this after-school latchkey ritual since he was about ten years old. He knows how to keep himself safe by not answering the door or letting anyone know that he is home alone. Steven likes this schedule, and Steven's mom feels confident that he can handle being alone in this way. She thinks it is helping him learn to be self-sufficient. But is it?

While it is important for kids to check in with parents, so their parents know where they are at all times, they still need the freedom to do things outside and explore within a set of boundaries. Steven's house acts like a plastic bubble, keeping him from the potential dangers of the outside world. If he were outside, he would be in great peril from strangers and the physical injuries that can come from skateboarding, bike riding, tree climbing, and all the other things that boys tend to do when left to their own devices. He may get into arguments with other boys or, even worse, his mother fears, engage in very dangerous behavior such as smoking or drinking. And what if he were to get abducted?

Parents today are fearful of allowing their children small moments of unsupervised time and even more fearful of allowing them to roam free with a roving gang of kids. We want to do all we can to keep them safe. Why, there are perverts and drug dealers out there, outside the plastic bubble of home. I often hear things like "The world is so dangerous today. So many things can happen." Well, the truth is that the world has never been safer. Children growing up in typical neighborhoods in the United States enjoy an incredible level of safety. Studies show they are not more likely to be abducted today than they were in previous generations. The truth is that the rate of stranger abductions has not increased, and it is possible that it has declined. However, due to the advent of global twenty-four-hour cable news networks, we see images of missing children near and far replayed over and over again each time it happens.

According to the 2005 NISMART report from the U.S. Department of Justice, there are only about 115 cases of child abduction in our entire country each year. Although this is 115 too many, it is certainly not the epidemic that many of us believe it is. Keeping our children indoors for fear of abduction by strangers is very much akin to keeping our children off airplanes for fear of a crash—which is very rare indeed—or out of cars for fear of an accident. Parents who really want to protect their children from harm should in theory keep them out of automobiles, right? That is where many, many children die each year. But of course, we would never do that. Our kids wouldn't be able to get to school or soccer practice or any of the other activities that teach them so much and help them grow.

The parents' challenge today is to recognize the many dangers of the world and to *equip their children to do the same* while instilling the confidence and self-reliance that are necessary to become independent, productive adults who live away from home. We can think of children, adolescents, and young adults as developing butterflies and take some cues from the metamorphosis that occurs from egg to caterpillar to flight.

The Caterpillar: Late Elementary through Middle School

I think of elementary and middle school as the caterpillar years. When the caterpillar larva is developing, it goes through four or five periods known as "instars." Every time it prepares to go into the next instar phase, it must shed its skin so that it may expand and grow. With each instar, the larva moves further and further from its place of origin in search of more food. Eventually, it begins the prepupal stage in preparation for the creation of the chrysalis. The caterpillar continues to wander until it finds exactly the right location to begin its metamorphosis.

School-age children, particularly those in middle school, need opportunities to shed their skin and find a safe place to begin establishing their identity. This is why young adolescents begin experimenting with their hair, clothing, language, and other forms of self-expression. They are discovering who they are and what they believe. They are learning to associate with others with whom they can identify and will even alter their own appearance to fit in with their crowd. This is how they stay safe emotionally. Similarly, caterpillars try to find a place to blend in with the environment to keep predators at bay as they are making the change into creatures capable of flight.

Parents must help their young caterpillars through what can be a very painful process, allowing their children to make mistakes and grow along the way. The following are some suggestions:

- Allow your child latitude with fashion and hair when possible. Learn his school's dress code, and establish standards of modesty within your own family. Outside of these rules and standards, allow your child to create his own identity through fashion. Don't get too hung up on hair and clothing. Hair grows back. Be stricter about things that will cause permanent changes to your child's body, such as tattoos or piercings. Anything short of that, within reason, can be healthy for your child to experience.

- Establish places where your child can develop independent mobility. For example, are there any stores or other public places where your child can ride his bicycle from your home? Help him set up excursions with his friends that don't require parental supervision. Teach him to stay in groups, as abductions are not likely when there are several kids together, and not to accept any rides or items from strangers. Equip him with a phone so he can call you when he gets to his destination and when he is on his way home.

- Encourage your child to take risks by requiring her to participate in a limited number of scheduled activities. You don't want to overschedule her (more about that in a later chapter). Have her try one new thing in sports and the arts each year so she can find a place to fit in and take risks. Ensuring participation in sports *and* the arts will help her explore lots of different things. Be sure she understands that she needs to commit to each activity she chooses, and require that she finish it. By doing so, you will be teaching your child the value of trying new things and providing her with built-in adversity that she must overcome.

- Face a new fear with your child. Go on a scary rollercoaster, or learn something new that you may have thought was risky before. Talk to your child about fear, and experience the joy in overcoming it together.

- Seek out a new adventure with your entire family. Try camping, scuba diving, rock climbing, or anything that would be completely out of the realm of your past experiences. Let your child watch you take risks and rise above adversity.

- Enroll your child in babysitting classes where he can learn first aid and CPR. These are offered through the Red Cross, the YMCA, and other community groups. Such classes help young people develop the confidence they need to take care of others who are younger and will help you feel more comfortable leaving your child home alone.

- Find ways for your child to have outdoor interaction with peers after school. You might be able to trade off days with neighbors to be home at that time. The middle school years are the most important time for you to be there when your child gets home from school. Ideally, a preteen should be able to move around the neighborhood with friends and bop in and out of the house for refreshments, to tell you a story, and so on. If you can't be there yourself, consider getting a neighbor to help or even hiring someone for this purpose. A college student who can function as more of a big-brother figure than a babysitter works well.

• Above all, never let your child give up anything just because it gets tough. Be very careful not to instill your fears into your child throughout this process. Yes, she will probably fail from time to time. She may become embarrassed or stressed or nervous or upset. But don't let her quit. A child who learns to finish things will learn tenacity and commitment. She will learn to get things done in school, on the job, and in life, regardless of the obstacles that are put in her way.

The Chrysalis: High School

High school is the time that many young people develop a kind of cocoon around themselves. Like the caterpillar, a teenager needs to be protected as he makes the transformation to adulthood. You may notice a change in your child's energy level at this point. By high school, the nonstop motion of the middle school years gives way to a more wary youth who tends to hide his face with his hair and to blend in as much as possible. You may notice that your child will have the same few friends and not want to venture into new groups. He may be careful about trying new things or experiencing anything that he may find uncomfortable or difficult. He may become fearful, not wanting to go far from home or even to drive a car.

On the whole, we have done a great job of teaching this generation the evils of hard drugs, drunk driving, and unprotected sexual intercourse. However, all the biological pulls of growing up are still there. As a result, recent studies have shown teens may be more likely to have oral sex with friends, not understanding that it can be even more dangerous than intercourse. They may huff on regular things found in the home, such as Magic Markers, and get high off of cold pills. They may not get driver's licenses at all but end up in cars with very irresponsible and fearless peers. Although we have been able to shelter them from certain dangers in the grown-up world, peer pressure is still a problem. We have taught them to avoid, not to cope.

Our job during the chrysalis stage of development is to equip our children with the skills to experience the outside world. We have to fight the urge to help them create a cocoon around themselves. Here are some ways to help your kids:

- Help them get a driver's license, even if they don't want one. Many parents fear allowing their child to learn to drive because of the accident risk or make the mistake of allowing the child to wait until he is "ready." The result is that kids are older than ever before they learn to drive because they are afraid. Then, often when that child finally receives a license, he is given the keys to his own car without a second thought.

    If you do not have access to public transportation, help your child understand that driving is a skill that he must learn. You will increase your child's desire for a license by not providing a chauffeur service whenever it is requested. If you are nervous about teaching your child to drive, pay for professional instruction. Many states now have mandatory waiting periods of up to one year between the permit and the license. If your state does not have this requirement, make it your requirement.

    Once your child is licensed, make the road to complete independence gradual. Do not give him his own car. Instead, allow him to use yours with increasing frequency. Having him run errands for you and make short trips to taxi younger siblings are great ways to increase his responsibility and decrease your workload. Every now and then, allow him to take the car to school or a social event, ensuring that you know who will be in the car with him. Consider installing a GPS system so you know where he is at all times. You can also get cameras or other devices to check on his safety and driving habits. Use this new technology to your advantage to teach him to be a responsible driver.

- During the summer, send your teen away from you. Find a camp, school trip, precollege program, or volunteer activity that will take your child away from you for a period of time. Start with a trip of a few days' duration, and advance to a multiweek program. Your child needs to learn to function without you. Trips and overnight programs will require him to take care of himself, with adult assistance when necessary, but without you hovering over him. These experiences provide a critical transition to adulthood. Get a detailed itinerary so that you know what your child will be doing. Be sure that adults who will be responsible for your child have been trained properly and subjected to background screenings to minimize risks.

- Require your child to volunteer or work for pay. These invaluable experiences will translate into many adult skills. Help him identify potential employers. Have him talk to friends who are working. Connect him with your friends who are managers or business owners. Have him ask the school guidance counselor about opportunities. Teach him how to approach local shops and restaurants and to fill out job applications. If you live in an area that has a shortage of these entry-level positions, look for volunteer opportunities. Teach your child to get a list of agencies through the local chamber of commerce, United Way, or local government. Explain that applying for volunteer jobs works the same way as paid positions. Role-play interviewing to reduce his anxiety. Help him keep up the search until he has found the right opportunity.

- Find ways to help your child become involved in school or community activities. Require that he do something each year to engage himself in the community. Check school and community Web sites to see what events might be coming up. Local festivals, art shows, and concerts are always looking for volunteers for just a day or two. Read the local paper together, and talk about ways to get involved. Talk about being part of the community and the kinds of things that might be fun to try. Consider things you both might do together. Think of things that might connect your child to his interests. For example, if he loves video games, see if the local electronics stores can tell you about gaming events. If he loves animals, maybe a local vet or animal shelter needs help.

- Require your child to do something new each year. This can be with you or on his own. It can be something simple, like drawing cartoon characters, or something as exciting as rock climbing. People with drive are always learning new things. They get interested in something and then go after it. Teens tend to avoid new things and need a little nudging. If your family expects everyone to do something new each year, your teen will learn the joy in experiencing something new. His fears will lessen with each new thing he tries. Have him talk to friends and teachers to get ideas. If he is stuck, take him to the local bookstore, and look at all the magazines devoted to specific activities.

- Engage your child in the performing arts, even if he is shy. Find a music group, play, or other activity that will require courage to complete. Most schools have a chorus or band. This might be a good place to start, since there is safety in numbers. Many places of worship have musical or drama groups for kids that can provide a nonintimidating environment to try the arts. You can also enroll your child in local recreation-center arts classes or find other less intense options.

The key in adolescence is to find lots of opportunities to try new things and meet new people. With each experience, your teen will gain the confidence and self-reliance necessary for success. He will also begin to understand what things excite and interest him.

The Emerging Butterfly: Post High School

As a butterfly emerges from its cocoon, it wiggles and wriggles until its exterior shell comes off. At first its wings look like little raisins, shriveled up and lifeless. But as it sits on the twig or wherever it was attached for its confinement, slowly its wings begin to fill with fluid. With each passing moment, the wings expand bigger and bigger until they begin to move gently. Finally, the butterfly becomes confident that its wings will carry it and takes flight in search of its adult life.

A young adult is kind of like the butterfly. She is not yet sure of herself. She needs to continually try to gain the courage necessary to fly away and lead an independent life. Your job as a parent at this point is to help her fill her wings with fluid so they will carry her away from you. The young adult is not quite ready to live on her own but needs to experience some independence. Here are some ways to foster this:

- If possible, have your child live in a dorm at college, rather than with you.
- If that is not possible, find ways to increase her independence while still living at home. Require that she work part-time and contribute to the family finances. Remember, the more you give her, the less she will need to earn. Therefore, you want her to contribute as much as possible. Also, encourage her to take trips to visit friends who are living at college.

- Talk about some of the family responsibilities she can take over, such as grocery shopping or cooking. Be very clear about her role in your household, and be sure she takes this responsibility seriously.
- Talk about her dreams for her future. Even if she doesn't know what kind of career she wants, she can probably tell you how she wants to live. Visit interesting places with her that may become her home someday. Talk about what type of education and career choices may enable her to live in those places.
- Help her get a vehicle, but require her to pay for its operation and maintenance. If she is on the family insurance policy, require her to pay her share.
- Treat her like the adult she is becoming, and be sure not to baby her.

Healthy Risks: Shaun White's Story

Shaun White is the amazing snowboarder and skateboarder who became one of the darlings of the 2006 Winter Olympics at age nineteen. He was born with a congenital heart defect that required two surgeries when he was very young. Many parents who have children with such serious heart problems shelter their children, afraid that each fall or stumble might result in tragedy. Shaun's parents did not do that.

When Shaun was only six, he decided he wanted to be like his big brother and learn to snowboard. Shaun's mother responded by contacting Burton, a company that makes snowboards, to find one that would be an appropriate size for her child. Shaun's dad quickly took up the sport so he could help Shaun learn and follow him around the mountain. Soon, however, Shaun was faster than his dad. Shaun's mother, in an effort to slow her son down a little, told him that he could only go down the mountain backward.

Instead of slowing down, Shaun just got faster going down backward. Shaun's parents understood that their son needed to take risks and to engage in life. Instead of telling him that he couldn't do dangerous things, they became involved in his sport and helped him train and improve, thus lessening the risk.

Millennial children have relatively few risks compared to the generations before them. We live in an affluent age with plenty of food, good health care, and lots of safety equipment. We can stay in constant communication with our children thanks to technology. Bikes and skateboards are safer thanks to helmets and padding. Children have become much more savvy about their own safety through education programs. Of course, nobody would suggest doing away with any of these things. However, there are ways to help children and adolescents (and even young adults) begin taking risks in their lives that will result in greater self-reliance and independence. We just need to take away the plastic bubble!

Once out of the bubble, your child needs to experience the normal pain and consequences that come from making mistakes and to use those experiences to learn and grow. Keep reading to learn how to encourage this process.

3. Decrease Rewards

Allow Life's Natural Consequences to Take Hold

Behind many teachers' desks sits the treasure box. It is filled with trinkets, candy, stickers, and little things that children in the classroom can pick when they have met the teacher's expectations for the day. During the 1970s and '80s, teachers learned the power of the treasure box and often used it to manage behavior in their classrooms. Even the toughest kids would suddenly get in line when a new cool toy was added to the teacher's arsenal.

The treasure box came about thanks to the work of Ivan Pavlov, B. F. Skinner, and other behaviorists of the twentieth century. Pavlov was a scientist who discovered that dogs could be conditioned to salivate when a bell rang. He did this by ringing a bell every time a dog was provided with food. After a while, the dog would salivate upon hearing the bell, even if there was not food present. Skinner also discovered that animals would engage in certain behaviors to receive rewards. Through various experiments, he developed theories of positive and negative reinforcement to entice humans to do things

71

to get something or to avoid certain consequences. Parents and educators throughout the twentieth century used this type of conditioning to get children to comply with their rules.

Behaviorists understand that children, like other creatures, will alter their behavior to achieve a desired result. The theory is if you do this, you will get that. Parents have long understood this phenomenon and used it to keep their children in line. Kids everywhere are rewarded through elaborate sticker charts on kitchen refrigerators. They earn actual money, or trips to McDonald's or ice cream parlors, or time on the computer. These types of rewards are known as *extrinsic motivators*. The idea is that eventually the child will begin to feel good by doing the right thing and do what is expected without the goodies. Doing the right thing because it is the right thing to do is called an *intrinsic motivator*. The ultimate goal in parenting is to get to that point. Intrinsic motivation is what spurs drive.

However, external rewards do not always lead to inner motivation. I see many parents today struggling with extrinsic motivators because their children don't seem to be able to move beyond such rewards. Children are so used to being rewarded for their behavior that they will say, "What will I get?" when told to do a simple chore such as making their bed or picking up their toys. Take six-year-old Lydia as an example. She lives in a very nice home with her parents and two brothers, and her room is like most American children's, with a huge closet filled with toys and clothes. There is a television mounted to her wall and a computer on the desk in the corner. She has at least ten Barbie dolls, loads of books, an iPod to listen to music, and every other item she has ever asked for. She has always been a pretty good kid, but lately her mother has noticed that she is talking back quite a bit.

Lydia's mom set up a behavior chart on the fridge to help Lydia alter her behavior. Every time her mom told her to do something and she did it without talking back, Lydia would get a sticker on the chart. When there were five stickers, Lydia would get a new outfit for her Barbie dolls. At first it worked really well. Lydia got five stickers, and her mom gave her a new outfit that she had bought ahead of time and stowed in her closet. By the end of the third day, however, Lydia had lost interest in the stickers. Her mom said, "Lydia, don't you want to earn another outfit for your Barbie?" Lydia replied, "I have enough outfits." Lydia's mom was stunned. None of the parenting books she had read informed her that Lydia wouldn't want the prizes.

Lydia's mom decided to use the time-out approach and move to negative reinforcement. Every time Lydia talked back, she was sent to her room for a time-out. But Lydia had no problem with this! Remember, her room was full of toys and electronics. Lydia's mom realized her error very quickly and changed the time-out area to a little corner of the kitchen. This, however, didn't seem to bother Lydia either. She did her time and then was free to go about her business.

Lydia's mom was using the all-too-familiar carrot-and-stick approach with her daughter. When Lydia did something good, she was fed a carrot, just as a trainer would give a horse. When she did something bad, she got the stick. The only problem was that Lydia's belly was already full of carrots, and she really couldn't feel the sticks. We live in a very affluent society where kids get a toy with every fast-food meal. Even children who come from families of modest means get the benefits of mass production and have loads of stuff. Meanwhile, the sticks parents use tend to be very gentle. When children are grounded, they retreat to bedrooms full of entertainment and electronics. Parents are often fearful of inflicting punishments that may result in their children not liking them.

For this approach to work, Lydia would need to become hungry again to appreciate the carrots and would need to feel the sting of much harder sticks. More important, Lydia's mom would need to help Lydia move quickly toward intrinsic motivators and doing the right thing because it is the right thing to do. Extrinsic motivators should not be used forever and are most effective when they are used randomly and sparingly. They should be discontinued as quickly as possible, when the child has learned the behavior.

Improving Your Child's Behavior

Every parent can incorporate a very simple four-step plan to improve behavior:

1. *Define the behavior of concern.* For example, Lydia talked back to her mother when told to do something.
2. *Determine why the child is engaging in this behavior.* There are four typical reasons a child will defy a parent in normal daily interactions. Assess which one is affecting your child:

   Power: "You can't make me."

   Attention: "Look at me! Look at me!"

   Control: "I want to do this now."

   Unmet physiological needs: "I am hungry/thirsty/tired/uncomfortable."
3. *Prevent the behavior by controlling the causes.*

   Power: Allow the child to make some minor decisions for the family (e.g., dinner and movie choices).

   Attention: Take a good look at how much quality time you spend with your child.

   Control: Find ways for her to be in charge of certain aspects of her life, and allow her to make certain decisions for herself.

   Unmet physiological needs: Ensure that she is getting proper nutrition, ample exercise, and plenty of sleep.
4. *Respond to the unwanted behavior.* Even if you do everything in your power to prevent unwanted behaviors, some will continue. Growing up means testing the boundaries and experimenting with cause and effect. Your child will try you again and again

before mastering each new skill. It's like *Survivor*—you must have the fortitude to outlast, outwit, and outplay your child.

When my daughter was only about three and a half, she started talking back to me. Every time she talked back, she was punished in some way, yet she continued. At the end of one particularly stressful day, I finally said to her, "Alison, you keep doing the same thing over and over, and you keep getting punished for it. Why do you continue to do this?" She looked at me square in the eye and said, "Because, one day, you'll get tired." I just sat there completely dumbfounded for a moment and then resolved that I would never get tired. I realized at that moment that my husband and I were in for quite an experience parenting a girl with such a spirit. I also realized that to have an impact, we would have to increase the severity of each consequence.

Power

Have you ever seen a Chihuahua walk up to a really big dog and bark? The Chihuahua doesn't seem to know how small it is and the kind of damage the big dog can inflict. It will stand there barking and barking unless the big dog asserts itself in a big way. The trouble is that some big dogs don't understand how big they are. They fail to use their power and sometimes get bossed around by little dogs.

By bossing their parents around, children who seek power are doing just what the Chihuahua does. Children who have the need for power should be given some. Allow your child to decide things for the family from time to time, such as what to have for dinner or where to go for fun on a Saturday afternoon. Let her make decisions for the entire family when you are content with either choice. Be sure to differentiate between daily decisions and life-altering ones. For example, kids may choose at which restaurant the family will eat or what movie they will watch, but you'd need the final say-so about which school your child will attend. Above all, do not invite your child to make a decision and then go against what she has decided. If you make this mistake, you will completely undermine her power, causing her to rebel even more.

Be sure your child understands that sometimes you will have to make key decisions because it is your job. Do not get into a tug-of-war. Just let your child know when you have complete power and when she can assume some. This is when it might be appropriate to say, "Because I am the mom and I said so." Your child needs to understand that you are absolutely in charge and that you relinquish power only at times when it is appropriate and healthy for all concerned.

Attention

Have you ever watched children at a playground or community pool with their parents? They will do trick after trick, shouting, "Look at me! Look at me!" The parents have to watch the whole time and provide the appropriate "Wow" or "That's great!" As soon as the parents take their eyes away for a second to have an adult conversation, the child will continue to pester until all eyes are on her again. Children absolutely crave attention, and it is your moral obligation as a parent to provide as much of it as you can. Many parents make the mistake of believing that the quality of time, and not the quantity, is important. Both are important. Different children crave different amounts of attention. The same child may crave more attention this week than she did the week before. It is critical to always be aware of your child's need for attention and to provide it as required.

Help Your Child Transition from School to Home
The transition from school and work to home each evening is typically the most difficult time of day. Parents have a thousand things on their mind. Sometimes they have to stop at the grocery

store or run other errands on the way home. By the time everyone gets home, there is dinner to be prepared, homework to be done, and many other things to attend to. This is always the time your child needs the most attention because she has not seen you for most of the day. It is also the toughest time to provide the required attention. But what most parents fail to understand is that the faster you provide the attention, the less time it will take. Most children are satisfied with a few moments of your time when you get home and then will go on and play. Instead of reading the mail or listening to your messages when you get home, start a ritual of sitting down with your child and hearing about her day. Younger children may want to play with you during this time; older ones may just want to talk. This debriefing typically takes only about fifteen minutes and is a great opportunity for you to learn about what is going on in your child's world: her friends, interests, challenges, and so on. Then you can do the things you need to do personally to unwind. The entire evening will go more smoothly, and unwanted behaviors will decrease.

Give One-on-One Attention
If you have multiple children, it is critical that you reserve special time for each one. The more children you have, the more vital this becomes. Spending one-on-one time with your kids becomes even more important as they get older and spend less time at home.

When my son was a senior in high school, he was out most of the time. It was very difficult to connect with him in any meaningful way. One Sunday, after a week when we really hadn't seen each other at all, we decided to go to a diner for breakfast—and to my surprise, he talked nonstop. This quickly became a weekly ritual. No matter what else was going on, we reserved Sunday mornings for our breakfast. Since we didn't really have the daily debriefing time anymore, he would save it all up for Sundays and unload everything that was on his mind. When he was in college, we continued this any weekend he was home or when I visited him at school. Even though we had less and less time together, we were able to invest in our relationship and keep it strong through this ritual.

Think about a time each week that you can reserve for one-to-one time with your child. It may be going to the mall or taking a walk or enjoying a sunset together. Create a ritual of your own and stick with it.

Set Limits on Technology

With the advent of cell phones, handheld devices, and e-mail, we are more in touch with others than ever before. While this can allow families to spend more time together, it can also diminish the quality of that time. Always remember that technology is there for you, not the other way around. Establish rules for your family to manage technology. If you are having a conversation, everyone must turn off his or her cell phone. If you are enjoying a fun activity together, put the handheld away for a while. If you must be connected with your office, provide your colleagues with clear instructions of what constitutes a real emergency. Set up times in advance of when you will be checking e-mail or voice mail. Talk to your children about how you manage the technology in your daily life, and require them to do the same.

Control

For a child, control can mean managing time. She wants to do what she wants to do when she wants to do it. If she is watching a video, she will normally want to see the end, even if she has seen the same video a dozen times. If she is playing with her toys, she will want to continue, even if it is time to go to bed. Control can mean deciding what she wants to wear, even if you don't seem to understand how important a particular brand name or style might be. Control is a little different from power. A child who seeks power wants to be in charge of you and other members of the family. A child who seeks control just wants to be in charge of herself.

The need for control is usually pretty easy to satisfy. A child who craves control needs to be offered choices and told the consequences of each one. The trick is to really allow your child to make those choices, even if you might consider one choice to be less advantageous than another choice. The SODAS method (developed by counselor Jan Rosa in 1973 at Boys Town, a home for troubled children) can be used to assist your child through the simple decision-making process:

Situation. Ask your child what is happening. Just say, "What's going on?" Stick to what and avoid asking why.

Options. Ask the child what his choices are in this situation.

Disadvantages. Ask him what unwanted things might occur for each choice.

Advantages. Ask him what desirable things might occur for each choice.

Solution. Summarize what he has determined are his choices and consequences, and then allow him to make a decision.

Unmet Physiological Needs

We've all seen the child in the grocery store who is whining, crying, or throwing a tantrum. Most of the time, the child is trying to communicate a need to the parent. The child may actually be hungry, tired, thirsty, too hot or cold, or uncomfortable in some way. Most parents are very skilled at interpreting the cries of their infant children but sometimes miss the cues of older children, teens, and even young adults. If your child starts to squawk, don't miss the opportunity to solve the problem quickly by providing what he needs at that moment. Be sure it is truly a *need*, as opposed to a want, and then satisfy this need to get the behavior under control.

Decreasing Rewards, Age by Age

Although the prevention strategies listed are effective in minimizing and responding to unwanted behaviors, you will still need some extrinsic motivators to help your child improve his behavior. The behavior theories from the early twentieth century still work, but a parent must make some adjustments for the youth of today.

The Defiant Middle Schooler

By the time your child reaches her middle school years, she already expects a prize for every completed school assignment and household chore. If your child doesn't respond unless there is a tangible reward, you have some work to do, depending on the situation at hand.

Household chores

- Choose your battles carefully. Many parents make the mistake of focusing on things that have no real consequences or meaning. Determine which things are nonnegotiable. If your child's room is messier than you would like, simply close the door. If she chooses to live this way, that is her choice. However, don't do things that assist her in dealing with the mess. If she loses a favorite article of clothing or important assignment, do *not* get in there to help her look. After the stress of the moment has ended, simply remind her that it is easier to find things in a clean room.
- Make your child completely responsible for things that impact her. She should be expected to do her own laundry; clean her own room, including dusting, vacuuming, and window washing; and clean her own bathroom, if she has one. Simply teach

her to do so, and then she is on her own. Don't harass her if it is not done, and don't bail her out when she doesn't have clean clothes to wear. She will learn quickly that she doesn't want to wear the same shirt more than once in a week! You will not need to provide any types of rewards or consequences; life's natural consequences will convince her to make the necessary changes.

- Make your child responsible for at least one task that is inter-connected to other tasks in the household. For example, make her responsible for setting the table for dinner, and don't put the food on the table until the table is set. You won't have to say a word; her hunger will eventually lead her to the cupboard to get the plates.

- If you have a pet, make her responsible for feeding it. The animal's demands for food will be much louder than your nagging.

School

- Do not attach rewards and consequences for grades. This is an area that is very difficult for parents. Many people (parents and educators alike) make the mistake of taking away sports and other activities when a child's grades go down. The theory is that the student would have more time for his studies if he weren't playing soccer. While it is important to have a healthy balance of activities (see chapter 6), taking away the things where the child is experiencing success is not the way to deal with lack of success in other areas. The middle school years are the time when a child finds out who he is and develops interests and passion in life. The last thing you want to do is take away the experiences that are so critical to his development.

- Focus on learning, not grades. Although middle school grades are important because they provide information to high school counselors and teachers about your child's abilities, they will not be viewed by colleges and future employers. These grades may not necessarily indicate how your child will do in high school and college. He doesn't necessarily develop the study skills in middle school that he will need in high school because he doesn't have the cognitive abilities to do so yet. In other words, lighten up about grades. Instead, focus on the learning. Focus on celebrating successes. Focus on identifying your child's interests and passions. Make school all about discovery and excitement.

- Remember what is truly important about learning during this time:
    - Learning is fun and a reward in and of itself.
    - Attendance is extremely important. Be sure your child goes to school on time every day. Don't give him mixed messages by scheduling vacations or appointments during school time.
    - Assignments should be completed on time. It is important for your child to meet the teacher's expectations, even when he doesn't agree with the assignment.
    - Encourage your child to take some new classes and to try everything he can in school.

Rewards

- Make rewards meaningful by not giving your child everything she wants all the time. You will need to curb the abundance in your life to reward your child appropriately (see chapter 7).
- Focus rewards on things that will require your child to contribute. If she wants a new cell phone, require her to pay half by completing tasks to get there.

Punishments

- Punishments need to be swift, severe, and complete. Many parents make the mistake of grounding for a week or a month and then giving in when the child whines loudly enough.

Instead, ground for just one day, but make it severe and complete. Don't allow your child any contact with the outside world. Cut her off from the computer, her cell phone, the TV, and all other forms of communication.

- During this time, keep her close to you by accomplishing a household chore together. Make it something difficult that will result in gratification at the end. Cleaning out the garage, weeding the garden, and painting are all good things you can do together. As you work, take advantage of the time together to drive your points home and strengthen your relationship.

Respect
- Always demand respect. The most important thing to remember, particularly with kids of middle school age, is that you are the parent. Your child should speak to you in a different manner than he speaks to his friends. Children generally start demonstrating disrespect in very small ways that tend to escalate as they get older. Of course, you must model this behavior yourself. Speak to him respectfully, and expect the same in return.
- Do not tolerate eye rolling, head tossing, or other physical gestures. Young adolescents are not always aware they are doing these things, so you must point them out. Explain to your son that he is in control of his body and is responsible for the messages he is sending by doing those things. If your son rolls his eyes, stop the conversation immediately and say, "Do not roll your eyes at me. That is disrespectful." Call him on this every time, and he will learn not to do it.
- Do not tolerate cursing, name-calling, or insults of any kind from your child. Again, stop him every time he does it, and require him to say things in a more respectable way.
- Do not tolerate it when your child uses a nasty tone of voice, raises his voice, or resorts to other audible signs of disrespect.

Stop him and imitate what he did so he will understand it. Have him repeat what he said using a respectful tone and volume.

- Do not allow him ever to walk away from a difficult conversation. Children of this age will often turn on their heels and run when you are telling them things they don't want to hear. Do not allow him to leave when you are speaking to him. Be sure he understands that you will decide when the conversation is over. If he goes to his room, follow him there and require him to come back to the room where you were talking. If he locks the door, explain that this is not permissible. If he continues to lock his door, remove it from its hinges and store it somewhere until he has learned to have civil conversations.

The Apathetic High Schooler

Adolescents can become quite apathetic during high school. Your job is to assist your child in continuing to care about something—anything—and stay on track in her development. You will need to continue using all the strategies listed for middle school students and add the following.

Driving. The car keys are your most powerful tool. If your teen is eager to drive, you have the ultimate behavior reinforcer: the car. However, many teens are now opting not to learn to drive (see chapter 4). If you live in an area where there is not ample public transportation—which is most of our country—then driving is a life skill that a productive adult must learn. It is critical to get your teen behind the wheel. To combat the reluctant-driver phenomenon, you have to stop driving your child to places she wants to go. The more inconvenient you make her life, the more she will desire to drive herself. Once your child can drive, do *not* give her a car of her own. Instead, let her use yours, provided she is doing what she needs to do. You can have her earn driving privileges through completing household chores, getting good grades, and so on. The keys to the car work beautifully, as long as she really needs them to do what she wants to do.

A budgeted allowance. Provide your child with a monthly allowance that is enough for her to buy only the essentials. Think about everything she will need, including clothing, cosmetics, shampoo, and school supplies. Then allow her to do her own shopping. If she buys clothes that are not appropriate for school, she will suffer. If she runs out of her favorite shampoo because she squandered her money on snacks, she will suffer. This will end the continual begging for money, will teach her to budget, and will provide her with a desire to work if she wants other things. (For more on this, see chapter 8.)

Once your child understands the limitations of her budget, provide her with opportunities to earn money or items. These opportunities can be simple, like doing the dishes, or challenging, like joining a new club at school.

A bright future. Help your child develop a vision for his future. However, don't expect that he will already know what he wants to do with his life. Instead, focus on life immediately after high school and his lifestyle in general. Take him to visit universities that have high academic requirements. Try to help him find a school that caters to things he is interested in. If he loves going to football games, go to a big state university where football is important. You might even try to get tickets to a game so he can experience it firsthand. If you live in a cold place and he loves to surf, find a school near the beach, and show him that acceptance to that school is his ticket to warmth, sand, and waves. Don't expect him to find relevance in the number of volumes in a school's library or in the academic rigor of its programs. Most high school students have no idea about the value of these things and cannot see past next week, let alone four years. Instead, really focus on the lifestyle he would find enticing, and exploit that. Once he's found a university that appeals to him, help him learn what kind of grades, test scores, and other requirements he will need to satisfy to get there. Then, when you find yourself battling over grades, you can remind him of what he is working toward.

The cost of things. Visit places where you think your child might ultimately want to live, and find out how much it will cost for her to live there. Visit model homes and talk about the price tags. Take test-drives in cars that she might like and talk about the cost. Help your child understand how expensive her wants are going to be, and talk about what she will need to do to earn the money to fulfill them.

Share your financial information with your child. If you are very well off financially, talk about times when you weren't and what it took to get where you are. It is essential that your child get a good sense of money and sacrifice for her to understand the rewards and consequences of behavior.

The Underachieving College Student

Establish expectations with your college-bound child. What kind of grades do you want him to get? First-year students should generally be expected to earn *at least* a 2.5 grade point average. This would be half Bs and half Cs, though you of course expect your child to do his best. By the second year, you should increase that minimum expectation to a 3.0, which would be half As and half Bs (or all Bs). Will you continue paying for tuition and other expenses if he doesn't meet these expectations?

You should determine just how many bad grades you are willing to subsidize ahead of time. Think of yourself as a scholarship program. Every scholarship program sets standards for grades to ensure it's not wasting valuable resources. Before the term begins, be sure that your child really understands what is expected. Talk about good work habits that will help him understand the material and get good grades. Talk about the temptations inherent in college that might distract him from studying. Sometimes it is a good idea to allow a student to continue for one more semester after failing to meet academic requirements. Together you can determine what caused the problem and take steps to remedy it. The uncertainty of being able to stay in college if one doesn't perform up to reasonable standards is often a huge motivator.

However, if the problem persists and grades and effort are still below par, you would be wasting your money, and your child's time, by continuing to finance this lack of progress. Help him consider other work and/or educational options to move him forward.

The Moocher Adult

OK, you didn't read this book soon enough, and now you have a moocher living in your house. Chances are, you have turned rewards and consequences upside down. Your child has not been motivated to achieve independence, yet as a result, she is being completely taken care of. This one is easy—make her life more difficult! The consequence of coming home is less privacy, less free time, and more work. Create a "lease" for living in your home. Specify everything that is important to you, including sleep and wake times, rules for visitors, and rent (covering the cost of food, entertainment, and gas if she uses your car). Treat her more like a boarder and be sure she abides by the house rules. If she cannot comply with the lease, then she will need to find another place to live.

The reason children come home and stay home as adults is because it is easy. You need to make it tougher. When your child chooses to live with you at this age, she loses control of her own life.

Of course, there are times when an adult child moves home in the midst of a crisis that is completely out of her control. You can be sensitive to this for a reasonable period of time, but work with her to come up with a plan for her to regain independence. If it turns into a mooching situation, then it will be time to get tough and get her out of your house!

Some adult children are living on their own but are still subsidized by their parents. For some, everything from rent to groceries is covered. For others, just when you thought you had them off economic assistance, another crisis occurs and you are writing checks again.

In general, providing long-term financial assistance for things your child should be paying for or dealing with himself will reduce his drive. If you are providing ongoing financial help, then you will want to get involved in the financial planning of your child's life, with the goal of him taking over these responsibilities. Sit down with him, and go over all the details of his income and expenses. If his expenses outpace his income, help him figure out how to make more money or spend less—or a combination of both. Together you can create a budget that allows him to consider your assistance for set expenses. For example, you might agree to pay for electric service. Take a look at the bills for the past year. (If individual bills are not available, you can usually contact the utility company and get this information over the phone.) Pay a set amount for this expense. If his bills are higher than what you agree to subsidize, he will be responsible for the difference. If he has been unreliable in the past in spending money as allocated, you might consider paying the utility company directly until he develops more responsibility.

Be sure to put an exit date on this assistance. Tell your child how many months you are willing to pay his electric bill, and then pull the plug as promised when the exit date arrives. You can use this same strategy for any economic assistance you are providing your child. Make a plan and stick to it. Your child will gain independence and feel good in the process.

Always remember that your job is to raise an adult. Many parents focus on raising children and simply managing behavior. The key to getting the behavior you want is to expect it and create an environment where your child will want to do the right thing.

In the next chapter, you will learn how to lessen your child's scheduled, programmed activities so that there is plenty of time to explore, create, imagine, and enjoy life.

4. Deschedule
Encourage Joy, Imagination, and Creativity

Mandy was so excited to be a new mom. She wanted to be sure that her child had the best life could offer, including every opportunity to try new things and really be involved in life. Even before her baby was born, she began his education by playing audio recordings of Mozart for him. As soon as Ryan was born, she started the Baby Einstein DVDs on the television. When he was just a few months old, she enrolled in a Mommy and Me class at the local community center. When Ryan turned one, she started him in preschool music and art. Once he was toddling, he enjoyed a creative preschool program three mornings a week, baby yoga one afternoon a week, and at least two playdates per week. By the time Ryan was four, Mandy decided he needed to be in a full-time academic preschool so he would be able to keep up with his kindergarten peers—and at the same time, enrolled him in swimming classes, a peewee soccer league, and Suzuki violin classes. Mandy became concerned about Ryan's academic progress, so she included a supplemental early-learning program, complete with its programmed workbooks, in her little boy's very busy schedule.

As her child grew, Mandy was always sure to keep him very busy. She spent hours on the road every day getting her son to each of his scheduled activities—including soccer, karate, piano, church youth group, supplemental tutoring, and horseback riding—to make sure that he was getting that important edge over other children.

Sound familiar? Mandy and Ryan were so busy that they ate fast food in the car at least twice a week and had no evenings or weekends without scheduled events. While it is very important for a child to take part in a wide variety of activities during their developmental years, too much of a good thing can rob them of drive. Usually, one or two scheduled activities at a time is plenty. If your child participates in competitive sports, limit it to one team per season. You can easily add one music lesson per week to this schedule, but you probably don't want to include being in a competitive dance team with three rehearsals per week.

Think of all activities as major or minor. A major activity includes more than two obligations per week, totals more than four hours of scheduled time commitment (including transportation to and from the activity), and is more than two weeks in duration. Examples of major activities would be sports teams, competitive bands and choruses, plays, and some religious instruction and youth groups. Minor activities require less of a time commitment and include things like piano lessons, tutoring, noncompetitive dance lessons, and noncompetitive karate lessons. At any given time, it is ideal for your child to have a maximum of one major and one minor activity. This will allow him to experience all life has to offer, but not all at the same time!

Too Much of a Good Thing

Mandy was raising an overscheduled child. She left no stone unturned to provide her child just the right experiences at just the right time, making sure each day was filled with a series of highly structured activities. She did not want to leave Ryan's learning and development to chance; she wanted to create the ideal environment for him to be smart, athletic, and creative. "I was concerned that my son would be lying around, so to keep him moving, I made sure he was always doing something," she said. Once he became a young teen, Mandy saw the error of her ways. Ryan complained about being bored anytime he had even a moment of unscheduled time. Yet he complained when he had to go to one of his programmed activities. He didn't seem to want to do anything.

"I can't understand why he refuses to join things and then complains that he has nothing to do. In school he has difficulty with subjects that require a lot of reading and note taking. He seems to want the teachers to entertain him all the time and doesn't understand how to be still," Mandy said. Ryan needed very direct instructions to get anything done. Halfway through a task, he tended to lose interest and would go to find something else. He often acted offended when Mandy tried to get him involved in family activities or other fun.

Mandy was worried that Ryan would not have any real interests or passions in life. So she started working hard to turn back the clock and teach him how to enjoy his own time.

Mandy's son suffered from a lack of imagination and the inability to find interest in anything. Children being raised in our modern world often suffer from this problem because they have always had their play and free time scheduled for them, from very young ages, and were not allowed to just be kids and discover their interests on their own. David Elkind, PhD, chronicled this phenomenon in his 2007 book, *The Power of Play*. Imagination, creativity, and the desire for discovery provide the fuel for drive. Without them, kids don't really want to do things or be things. Some parents, like Mandy, think they are giving their children an advantage by providing them with lots of programmed activities. Other parents are forced to do so because of work schedules.

The truth is that children need a healthy balance of planned, programmed activities *and* time to just be kids. Their imaginations flourish when they are given the time and space to grow. Creative thinking is only possible when the mind is idle for a time. Think about when you have had your best ideas. Was it when you were busy doing things and thinking about things, or when your brain was less active? I get my best ideas in the shower, during a walk, or following a Sunday afternoon nap. If you really need to figure out how to solve a problem, do you make sure you have lots of structured things happening, or do you try and clear your head through some type of relaxation? Some corporations have created work environments around this idea. Microsoft, Apple, Google, and other high-tech companies have campuses where workers can walk, exercise, play, eat, and enjoy time together as they engage in the creative process. These companies have highly flexible work schedules so people can make time for what is important to them. They depend on employees who are driven and productive and ensure their work environment encourages that.

So how much is enough, and how much is too much? While there is no one answer for every child, there needs to be a balance. If your child doesn't have time each day when he doesn't have to make his own fun or just "be," then he is too busy. If your child complains often that he is bored, he is probably suffering from overscheduling. If your child is unable to sit in the car without the entertainment system going, he may have difficulty paying attention in school.

If you overscheduled your child when he was younger and are now wanting to make a change, it is not too late. Start by doing some things together with your teen that are not scheduled or structured. Try browsing in a bookstore or enjoying some time in a coffee shop together on a lazy Saturday afternoon. Go for a walk in the woods, and see how many different birds you can find. Lay in the grass in your backyard, and find pictures in the clouds. You will need to do these things together at first so your teen will get the idea. Slowly reduce the amount of scheduled time, and fill it with unstructured activities that you can do together. Your teen will soon learn to enjoy these things on his own.

What Is Programming?

Now that you have the quantity of activities under control, you can start considering the quality. Some types of activities encourage kids to explore, discover, and create, while others just make kids follow directions. You want to limit programming your child whenever possible. When a computer is programmed, it is "taught" to respond exactly the same way every time you give it the same types of instructions. Computers must be programmed by the user to do everything they are expected to do. If you give your computer instructions it has not seen before, it will not respond in any meaningful way and may even crash in the process. People, unlike computers, are capable of multiple responses to the same requests, can change their responses at any time, and respond to new situations in meaningful ways. Children need to develop this ability. However, if they are given explicit instructions and told exactly how to react each time, they will not learn to respond in meaningful ways to new conditions and may even "crash" in the process. Unfortunately, many parents believe that the more they program their children, the smarter and more able to function the children will become. It doesn't work that way. Children must be encouraged to make decisions, imagine, and make their own fun to develop the skills that are essential to independent functioning.

Recently in my school, a student named Ariel was sent to the main office by her teacher to make some copies. I happened to be in the vicinity of the copier as she was attempting to complete her task. She put the originals in the feeder and pressed the button. The copies came out in the right spot, but the paper was blank. She said to me, "I am going back to class. The copier isn't working. I guess it needs toner." I told her to go back to the copier and figure out what the problem was. Ariel looked at the screen and did not see any instructions; she repeated that the copier wasn't working and attempted to go back to class again. I asked Ariel to try and figure out what the problem was. She got quite distressed and told me that she had never had any copy machine classes and simply did not know what was wrong. Finally, I went with Ariel and asked her to repeat exactly what she had done on the copier. It turned out that she had placed the originals in the feeder upside down. Ariel is a student who has great difficulty solving simple problems. She is a wonderful person who wants to succeed. However, she must be given explicit instructions to complete tasks. It is important that young people are given opportunities that require them to engage in creative problem solving so they can develop this important ability.

Someone who is driven sees possibilities before him and works to move toward those possibilities. This cannot be done without the ability to think independently. Be sure to provide your child, teen, or young adult with an environment that encourages and requires him to use his brain to learn and solve problems. There are many factors that must be in place for this to happen:

- A thoughtful balance of structured activities and free time
- A calm environment with limited stimuli
- A peaceful start and end to each day
- Good nutrition

- Fresh air and exercise
- The requirement to make decisions in everyday life
- Participation in activities and events that demand independent thinking

In other words, the brain needs to be given the context in which to function properly and allowed to program itself. A brain that is continually directed and structured will do only what the external programming teaches it to do. It becomes lazy and unable to make the constant connections necessary to learn. People who are driven are constantly moving forward—going over, under, and around obstacles. If one way doesn't work, they try another way and another and another until they get where they want to go. If we continually tell our kids how to do everything, they learn that there is only one way: the way they are told. They need opportunities to figure things out on their own, developing multiple solutions to problems.

A highly functional brain should act almost like an old-fashioned pinball machine. Each idea is like the ball, propelled by an impact from an external force. It rolls up into the main chamber of the machine and bounces off each wall. From time to time, it will rest on a spot for a moment and then be launched in a completely new direction. Just when you thought it was done, it gets hit by a paddle and launched all over again. Bright children and adults with highly functional brains make unexpected connections between seemingly unrelated items. Their brains are always searching, reaching, learning. As parents, we must provide the proper context for these connections to happen, encouraging the spheres of ideas to bounce around as if in a pinball machine, lighting up and making sounds with each touch.

Let's take a young teen named George as an example. George had a homework assignment that required the use of his math textbook. George began doing his homework after dinner and soon discovered that he did not have the book. He got very upset because he knew he would have detention the following day if he failed to complete the assignment. This was an excellent opportunity for George to practice problem-solving skills. Here is how each type of parent might handle this situation:

Helicopter parent. This parent would write a note to George's teacher, explaining that the family was very busy and that George did not have time to get the work done. This parent would either e-mail the teacher, call the school, or have George bring the note in. If the teacher did not accept the excuse, this parent would become irate, accusing the school of not being fair to her child and family.

Hot air balloon parent. This parent would not worry about it—it's just one math assignment—and likely show up at the regular time the following day to pick up George. What teacher would give detention over a single uncompleted homework assignment?

Pathfinder parent. This parent would talk with George and ask him to think of some things he could do to solve the problem. She would brainstorm with George about some strategies, asking some key questions. Who could you call for help? Can you e-mail the teacher? Does the class have a Web site with more details? Is there any way to get the book from someone else? Do you have the problems written somewhere else? What kind of problems are they? Could we make up some other problems that are similar so that you can at least practice what the teacher wants you to practice? This parent would keep talking with George until he determined the best solution to the problem. If there was no solution that George could find, she would help him understand that he would need to accept his punishment of detention and use this as an opportunity to learn.

This type of problem solving must be learned through continual experience. Only then is a young person able to see far enough ahead to desire to propel his life forward.

The Deprogrammed Child

What does a deprogrammed child look like? When Gavin was seven years old, he was always in his own little world, the one he created for himself. He frequently raided the kitchen cupboard for a metal colander to serve as a helmet of sorts. A wooden spoon became a paddle for an imaginary boat that he made out of a laundry hamper. Gavin's mom often was an unwitting accomplice in the stories he created. There were villains to be fought, evil forces to be destroyed, and battles to be won. As Gavin grew, he no longer lived in this world. Little by little, the kitchen items found their way back to the cupboards, and his fantasy life faded away. As a preteen, he would ride his bike around the neighborhood with friends. Sometimes they would stop and lay on the grass looking up at the clouds, creating pictures in their minds with the changing shapes. During long summer evenings, they would tell scary stories and stupid fart jokes. When Gavin became a teenager, he would lie on his bed for hours, just listening to music. His parents assumed he was napping, but he was actually awake and very engaged. Sometimes he was dreaming about the new girl he had met or his life as a professional ballplayer. Gavin loved this time alone when he could get lost in his thoughts. It seemed to give him the energy and creativity to try new things. Gavin never got bored because he loved to read, draw, and hang out with his friends.

As Gavin got older, he had no idea what he wanted to do with his future. He loved to do so many things that he could hardly narrow it down to one. He looked forward to college and moving out of the house. Gavin's balanced life as a child allowed him to imagine his future and enjoy life with every step toward adulthood.

Distractible Middle Schoolers

Young adolescents have brains that change direction at a moment's notice. Just when you think they are about to string two thoughts together, they go in a completely different direction. Their emotions easily escalate, making everything a crisis. When dealing with children of this age, you have to continually determine whether they are functioning as little ones or teens because they go back and forth so frequently. Although this can be a frustrating age for parents, it is also wonderful. Your children still retain the joy, energy, and spontaneity of younger childhood days yet are beginning to develop the insight of a more mature age. Use the following strategies to keep middle schoolers' young, flexible minds on track:

- *Balance structured activities and free time.* Be sure that your child's daily schedule includes at least one to two hours of unstructured time that isn't screen time (i.e., television, texting, or computer time). Have one free day per week for your child.

- *Provide a calm environment with limited stimuli.* Continually evaluate how much screen time your child has daily. Limit that time to no more than about two hours per day. Do not allow your child to have a television, computer, gaming system, cell phone, or other technology in his bedroom. Have a place in your home where these items are "checked in" each evening. Secure your Internet so that your youngster can access it only when you say it is OK.

- *Teach your child to prepare for the next day.* At this age, the start of each day actually occurs the night before. Talk about what is going to be happening the following day. Get backpacks, supplies, lunches, and so forth together and ready as much as possible. Determine how much time it will take to get ready, including ample time for a sit-down breakfast. Get your child an alarm clock, and teach him to use it. Avoid fights about getting up in the morning by teaching your child to be responsible for himself—if he doesn't wake himself up, he will miss his ride. Sit down with your child at breakfast, or at least be in the kitchen talking with him as he eats his cereal. Review what you will be doing during the day. Most important, do not have the television or talk radio on during this time. Play music that promotes healthy brain activity, such as classical or jazz.

- *Promote good nutrition.* The importance of good nutrition cannot be stressed enough. Many children at this age are surviving only on sugar. Be sure you provide healthy options that include fat, protein, and complex carbohydrates in balance. Middle schoolers' developing brains require fat and protein. There is a theory that high amounts of sugar promote high activity in children. Much research has disproved this myth. One of the biggest problems with a high-sugar diet is what kids are *not* eating. If they are filling up on soda and junk food, they are not eating nutritious foods that allow them to grow, learn, and focus. Really pay attention to what your child is eating, and control this as much as you can. Many schools can provide you with details of what your child is eating at school. You can absolutely influence what your child eats in your home by providing only the healthiest options. Don't worry when your child is out with friends or if he trades lunches occasionally. As long as you supervise the meals within your control, he will be just fine.
- *Encourage fresh air and exercise.* Preteens and young teens need lots of time and opportunity for free play outside. Be sure they can skateboard or ride bikes or swim or run around every day. They are still young enough at this age to enjoy a playground or a game of tag. Encourage, and even require, them to play outside with their friends each day.

- *Require kids to make decisions in everyday life.* Provide lots of opportunities for your child to make decisions. Deciding between dinner options, picking out clothing, assisting in choosing a vacation or outing destination are all examples of ways kids can learn to make decisions at this age.
- *Choose group activities and events that demand independent thinking.* These activities include reading, performing arts, gardening, Odyssey of the Mind (this is an international problem-solving competition; see www.odysseyofthemind .com), and visual arts—all great options for this age group.

Fatigued High Schoolers

As young people move into the teenage years, they tend to become less energetic. They need strategies comparable to those appropriate for their younger counterparts, with just a few adjustments:

- *Balance structured activities and free time.* Teens should begin to gravitate toward one or two things that interest them at this point. Help your teen find what really interests him, and encourage him to stick with it. At this age, more competitive activities are appropriate. However, be careful to still include some unstructured time, at least two or three days per week, and one large chunk of time once per week when your teen can relax.
- *Limit screen time.* Continue regulating screen time for your teen. A maximum of two hours per day on the computer, in front of the television, texting, and gaming should be your goal. However, be aware that homework loads at this age may require more time in front of the computer. You will need to be diligent at monitoring this. Keep technology out of your child's bedroom to help him establish a normal sleep schedule.

- *Require teens to get up for school on their own.* It is essential that teens be completely responsible for getting up on their own and getting ready for the day. If you did not require your teen to use an alarm clock in earlier years, be sure to start right away. You *must* get out of the habit of getting him up and moving. Teens tend to become nocturnal. You must do all you can to work toward a normal wake/sleep cycle. Help him avoid caffeine in the evenings, and develop a routine that allows for relaxing activities after dinner. Video games make the brain accelerate and should be avoided in the evenings to help prevent sleep issues. These games also make the brain highly distractible and should be avoided in the early-morning hours as well. Limit gaming time to the late afternoons to avoid these problems.

- *Be sure your home is fairly calm and quiet in the mornings.* If you like to listen to music in the mornings, try classical; if your kids don't like that, allow anything that is melodic with appropriate language. Avoid abrasive heavy metal or rap.

    Spend at least a few minutes with your teen in the morning, ensuring that you both understand the plan for the day. Provide him with encouragement to meet any anticipated challenges, and help him ensure that he is ready for the day.

- *Promote good nutrition.* Control the food that is in your home. Be sure to have lots of healthy options available, and reduce the amount of junk food in your cupboards. Teens generally eat enormous amounts of food. They will gravitate toward things that are easy and full of simple carbs and sugar. Cereal and sandwiches tend to be their favorites. Put attractive fruit in a bowl on the counter. Keep cheese sticks and healthy microwavable items handy. Be sure you have a plan for dinner each evening that includes healthy foods. Then don't worry about the rest. You will have very little control over what your teen eats outside the home. Just do as much as you can in your own home.

- *Encourage fresh air and exercise.* Teens will need a little more prompting to get out into the fresh air. If your child doesn't have much interest, you might have to lead the way. Require your teen to walk the dog—or even walk you! Establish a daily walking ritual, and require him to accompany you and/or the dog. Start a new hobby together, such as bike riding or a sport that gets you both outside.

- *Require teens to make everyday decisions.* Your teen should begin making more and more important decisions so that he is prepared for the really big life choices. Have him pick his classes for school. Give him a monthly budget that includes money for clothing, entertainment, and toiletries. And don't bail him out when he makes mistakes.

- *Require participation in activities and events that demand independent thinking.* Your teen can start doing volunteer work or paid work. He can continue his involvement in performing and visual arts, enter creative-writing contests, work on school newspapers, enter robotics competitions, or participate in other types of things that require lots of thoughtful involvement.

Jaded Young Adults

If you didn't lay the groundwork earlier, you may have a special challenge on your hands with your young adult child. By this time, a young person without drive has permanently parked himself on your couch and doesn't seem to want to move at all. Instead of worrying that you are structuring his life too much, you must require that he do *something*. Now you need to get tough. You will need to establish very clear house rules that he must follow to retain his right to reside with you.

Rule 1. It is your *house.* You determine your house schedule, when lights-out occurs, and when everyone must be up and out of bed.

Rule 2. A couch is not a bed. All residents must sleep only in their beds, only at designated times.

Rule 3. Every adult resident is responsible for waking and rising on his own. You are not to get your child out of bed.

Rule 4. Again, it is your house. You determine when the television and other stimuli can be on.

Rule 5. Have family meals in the evenings, with a designated dinner time. If your young adult wants dinner, he must appear at the designated time. Otherwise, he is on his own. At this point, you will want to limit convenience foods and keep only things that need to be prepared. This will help you control the consumption levels of your adult child and his friends.

Rule 6. Every member of the household must contribute to the care and upkeep of the home.

Living in Balance

A child who is told what to do and how to do it every moment of the day is being pushed along through life. Drive comes from having to move oneself without someone pushing or pulling. A child with drive sees something he wants to do and goes for it. It is important, however, for children to get exposed to many different things so they can see the infinite possibilities in life. This exposure is critical—to a point. It must be within the context of a well-balanced home life and schedule. Too many activities can create a life that is out of balance and actually rob a child of drive.

A family should have a sort of rhythm, allowing each member to move forward at a consistent, steady pace. From time to time, the pace will quicken as one or more family members engage in important short-term projects or approach critical deadlines. If your family feels frantic most of the time, there is something wrong, and you need to restore balance. Here is a sample schedule that would be typical of a family in balance:

6:00 a.m.—Mom gets up and gets ready for work.

6:30 a.m.—Dad and kids get up and talk to Mom for a few minutes.

6:45 a.m.—Mom leaves for work. Dad and kids eat cereal together and then get ready for the day.

7:30 a.m.—Dad and kids leave the house for work and school.

3:30 p.m.—Mom picks the middle school child up at school. Mom and the middle schooler go home for a snack and to do homework. The high school child stays at school for soccer practice, which occurs four to five times a week for about three months.

5:00 p.m.—Dad picks up the high schooler and brings him home.

5:30 p.m.—The family has a quick dinner together.

6:00 p.m.—Mom takes the middle schooler to play rehearsal, which takes place twice a week at the community theater. Mom takes the opportunity during play rehearsal to get caught up on her e-mail and read. The high schooler assists Dad with the dishes and then does homework.

8:00 p.m.—Mom and the middle schooler return. The family watches a little bit of television. They talk a bit about the day and the following day's schedule.

Of course, things get more hectic from time to time. During the play's actual production time, the middle schooler must be at the theater every night. This happens to fall during the same week the high schooler's soccer team is in the state championship play-offs. So Mom and Dad must split their time between the two events. After that week ends, the family has a week without any special activities and enjoys the time to just relax.

Unfortunately, many families have a schedule that involves multiple children involved in multiple activities simultaneously. Parents run from activity to activity, eating in the car and not really having any time to talk with one another. Children never have a moment to relax, to imagine, to just "be." At a minimum, arrange your family life to include the following:

- Time at the beginning and end of the day to connect with one another
- At least one evening a week when everyone is home together
- At least one day each week when each person has no obligations (these can occur on different days)
- Time built into each child's day when there is nothing on the agenda (the younger the child, the more time is needed; be sure you require your children to entertain themselves during this time)

Mandy's son Ryan is now fifteen. For the past couple of years, she has been using the strategies discussed in this chapter. Ryan is a different kid. He now has a band and is playing at community functions. He gets up by himself for school every day and usually gets his homework done without prompting. Ryan is starting to talk about college and seems to be excited about the future.

At first Mandy was concerned about making these changes. She was worried that people would think she wasn't a good mom because she made her son get up on his own in the morning and no longer harassed him to do his homework. And Ryan had trouble at first. He was late to school several times, and some of his grades fell. But he soon discovered what he had to do and began succeeding more than he ever had before. The best part of this transition for Mandy is her new relationship with her son. She is able to connect with him more and understand him better. Now that she is not orchestrating his every move, she can really pay attention to him as a thinking, feeling human being.

Applying the strategies in this chapter may seem overwhelming. Just try one little thing at a time. Once you have it mastered, move on to the next one. In a very short period of time, you will be able to transform your home into one that promotes drive in your child.

5. Reduce Comfort

*Counteract the Immense Abundance and
Indulgence of Our Culture*

Imagine sitting in a chair on the beach on a beautiful day. The temperature is about seventy-eight degrees, and a hint of a cool breeze is blowing on your face. You sink your toes into the sand as the umbrella shades you just enough to read your favorite book. In the distance, you see sailboats cruising by and graceful birds diving for fish. You are lulled by the sound of the waves gently rolling onto the shore. Nobody is demanding your attention, and you can relax in the moment. When will you move from this spot? Only when something disrupts you.

You aren't likely to leave the beach, or even be motivated to shift in your seat, until you feel uncomfortable. You might feel a sudden attack from mosquitoes, or you may need to go to the bathroom. Perhaps you are hungry or thirsty or begin to feel the first heat of sunburn. Maybe your young child starts to cry or argues with his siblings. The discomfort from these events will eventually drive you out of your chair and eventually off the beach altogether.

Discomfort causes movement and change. For a person to desire a change, he must feel uncomfortable. In modern America, we have created a world of extreme comfort for our children. But the very culture designed to make our children's lives easier actually has the opposite effect in the long run. It is difficult to have a fulfilling, happy adulthood when you don't know how to change and grow or how to go about getting what you want on your own. We need to encourage our kids by providing enough discomfort to create the drive that is essential to success in their adult years. Even if your child is already a young adult who is still living in your house, you can use discomfort to help him get on his way to a wonderful future (in his own house!).

How Did We Get to This Point?

Modern innovations and a strong American economy have provided amazing things to make our lives more comfortable. Children have benefited from the abundance and affluence of our culture. As they grow, their bedrooms become more and more like full-fledged entertainment zones, complete with computers, gaming systems, televisions, and music players just for them. They are chauffeured in vehicles to school, activities, lessons, and social events—never asked to walk or ride their bikes for fear that a stranger may take them. Many are not asked to perform chores. Their homes, vehicles, schools, and other facilities of interest are air-conditioned and heated to the perfect temperature all the time.

From the moment they are born, we do everything we can to keep them serene and feeling good. Believe it or not, modern potty training is a great example of how comfort, for the parent and child, has delayed learning and development. In the 1950s, the average age for potty training was eighteen months. Today, it is two years.* It is

---

* Michelle Quinn, "Life of the Potty," *San Jose Mercury News*, February 8, 2005, 1A.

very common and accepted in our culture to see children who are three or four still in diapers. The delay in training can be very stressful for families, day care, and educational providers. Children are at risk for diaper rash and infection and may even refuse to completely potty-train later. This is known as "stool refusal" and can result in constipation and even rectal impaction.* The longer it takes for a toddler to get out of diapers, the more diapers will end up in our landfills, adding to our concerns for the environment.

The advent of disposable diapers has, in part, prompted this delay. Parents don't have to wash cloth diapers and can go longer without having to change a diaper. Children feel dry even when they are wet, thus reducing the feeling of discomfort. The manufacturers have gone along with the trend, making larger diapers that have cute cartoon characters and pull-ups that look similar to big-kid pants. Since children can't feel any wetness, we now have diapers that change colors when wet and alarms that sense wetness while a child sleeps.

The stroller population is also becoming much older. It has become common for parents to use strollers with their children until almost kindergarten. Seeing this trend, manufacturers complied by making larger and more luxurious models. Parent and child comfort increased. Newer models include toys, cup holders (for parent and child), and ergonomic designs. Who would want to give this up? The benefit for the child is complete comfort; the benefit for the parent is assured safety and control. It is much easier to push a stroller than to monitor the movement of a curious toddler or preschooler. This phenomenon is chronicled in Nancy Lieberman's novel *Admissions*, set in an upscale private school in New York City. The protagonist describes parents of a five-year-old in a stroller by saying, "It had never occurred to them to venture into the world

---

* Bruce Taubman, "Toilet Training and Toileting Refusal for Stool Only," *Pediatrics* 99, no. 1 (1997): 54–58.

with their children free to move about. It seemed so risky, so dangerous, so inconvenient."*

The family vehicle has also become a very comfortable place to be. A recent minivan commercial shows two young boys sitting in their rear captain's chairs while the van is parked in the driveway. They are watching a DVD. Their father approaches and pleads with them to come to the cool new tree house he has just built in the backyard. One of the boys asks if it has air-conditioning or a DVD player. When the dad says that it does not, the boy responds, "We're good here." Typical children ride in style in large SUVs and minivans with rear climate controls, entertainment centers complete with their own controls and headphones, cup holders, snack trays, and automatic doors. Their belongings are safely stowed in the rear cargo area so they have plenty of space. Each child has her own seat and plenty of room. It is not unusual to see children reluctant to leave the comfort of the vehicle to go to school or back into the house.

Potty training, strollers, and family vehicles are only a few examples of how creature comforts have delayed developmental milestones and interfered with a child's ability to develop drive. Just as you would not want to move from the peaceful place on the beach, a child wants to maintain a comfortable status quo. Although any single example is seemingly innocuous, you can find many more examples simply by looking around. How is your home environment different from where you grew up? How have retail stores, movie theaters, grocery stores, and doctors' offices changed? Look around and you will find countless examples of wonderful comfort that permeate our culture and, when added together, create an environment that robs a child of opportunities to grow and develop.

* Nancy Lieberman, *Admissions* (New York: Time Warner Book Group, 2004), 231.

So What Can We Do Now?

If you are reading this book, you are probably the parent of an adolescent or young adult who lacks drive. Obviously, you can't go back and make your child walk without a stroller at age two or give him cloth diapers to encourage potty training. But don't despair. There are many ways to use discomfort, no matter how old your child is, to urge him to move and achieve.

The Unmotivated Middle Schooler

Christian is a typical seventh grader who loves video games and sending text messages to his friends on his cell phone. According to his parents, he does OK in school but is really not interested in anything. He is beginning to develop close friendships with a group of boys who all tend to dress the same, talk the same, and walk the same. Developing an identity and feeling like part of a group become extremely important at this age. Emerging adolescents will do almost anything to fit in.

Christian is home alone most afternoons and for much of the summer because both his parents work. But to pass the time, he is usually in front of a screen playing a video game, messaging his MySpace pals, or watching TV. When his dad gets home at about five, Christian tries to look busy doing his homework, but he doesn't usually get it all done on time.

He has a list of chores that he is required to do each week to earn his allowance. Sometimes he does them and sometimes he doesn't, but Christian gets paid anyway. If you ask him what interests he has, he will tell you that he likes to hang out with this friends, go to the mall, and play video games.

It's time to develop drive in Christian. This is actually the easiest age of life to do it. Middle schoolers have lots of energy and are still willing to try new things—if you insist. Use the following steps to bring your child out of his current state of comfort and turn his newfound discomfort into drive:

- Take your child's creature comforts away, and require him to earn them back one at a time. Instead of providing an allowance, have him work to earn specific things that he wants. Remind him that you own everything and only allow him to use what you think he should have at the moment. For example, he can earn a half hour of video-game time by mopping the floor. He can earn a movie on Friday night with his friends by cleaning out the garage. Don't worry what each item costs. Middle schoolers have difficulty understanding monetary relationships. For example, a cell phone is relatively inexpensive from a monetary standpoint, but it is invaluable to a twelve-year-old. Have your child make a list of the things that are most important, and negotiate with him on the value of each one. Be sure to have him make the list before he knows what you are up to so he won't artificially skew the values.

- Try and rework your schedules so that someone is home after school as much as possible. Whenever your child is too comfortable on the couch, get him up and moving. Require him to play outside until dinnertime.

- Have him transport himself whenever possible; don't hop in the car anytime he wants to go somewhere. Walking or bike riding are the preferred modes of transportation at this point, whenever safely possible. Find ways for him to travel in groups, and arm him with a walkie-talkie so you can communicate with him along the way.

- Require him to do his own laundry. He will only feel the discomfort of not having clean clothes once or twice before he figures this one out! This lessens your load and increases his independence.

- Don't interfere with the cleanliness (or lack thereof) of your child's room unless absolutely necessary. Allow him the discomfort of losing things and living in the mess. Just close the door if it offends you. He may not figure it out now, but he will eventually decide he wants to live in a cleaner environment. This may not happen until after he leaves you, but you are setting the stage for adulthood. The cleanliness of an adolescent's bedroom frequently becomes a power struggle and is really less important than so many other things. Choose not to have this battle!

- Make sure your child has a role in your family. He should be assigned certain jobs that impact others. These tasks are not to earn money or other things, as described earlier. They allow him to learn the discomfort of interrupting family life. For example, if his job is to clean the dishes and he fails to do it, the person who has to cook dinner the following night will suffer. He will have to rush and get it done so dinner can be made, or maybe the other person will have to cook dinner and work around the mess.

- Consider some very literal ways to connect creature comforts with monetary considerations. For example, don't use the air-conditioner in the car. Explain that gas has become very expensive and that it is much cheaper to run the car without it. If your child complains, ask him what he is willing to contribute or sacrifice to use the air-conditioning. (This strategy can be used with any creature comfort.) Or take him camping so he can experience life without creature comforts. Middle schoolers need very clear, literal examples to get the point.

- Get your child involved in after-school activities. Most communities have things for this age group to do. He may protest at first but will soon get used to it. Help him identify the possibilities. Let him know that you want him engaging in some productive activities with friends, and then help him select something that he might like. If he is quite comfortable being at home alone with all his gadgets and idle time, require that he try one new sport and one new arts activity each school year, so that he can explore all that life has to offer, until he finds one he likes. Don't allow him to quit, no matter how much he complains. Require him to finish what he starts.

The Directionless High School Student

Sarah is a high school freshman who doesn't really care much about her grades. Although she is very bright, she is satisfied with a C and rarely strives for more. So far, she really doesn't want to go away to college and doesn't have any real career goals. She figures she will just take a few community college courses and maybe work a little and then figure things out. Bob and Mary, her parents, aren't really worried. They see many other parents who have children like this, and those kids seem to figure things out eventually. After all, Sarah is only a freshman and still has over three years to go, so there's still plenty of time for her to find a direction. And either way, they think it will be fine for her to stay home for two or more years after high school. They certainly don't want to pay for her to go away to college if she doesn't have the motivation. It will sure save them a lot of money! So they are going to leave Sarah alone for now and see what happens.

In my view, Bob and Mary are making a huge mistake by allowing Sarah to coast through high school. Not only are they limiting her options after high school; they are inadvertently increasing the possibility that Sarah will drop out of high school! Nationally, the high school graduation rate is a stunning 71 percent. That means that 29 percent of students drop out.*

---

* Jay P. Greene and Marcus A. Winters, *Public High School Graduation and College Readiness Rates*, 1991–2002 (New York: The Center for Civic Innovation at the Manhattan Institute and The Bill and Melinda Gates Foundation, 2005), 7.

Students get very comfortable in their high school environment, enjoying the social stimulation and attachment to their friends. And the situation becomes more and more comfortable as they progress through the four years of high school. Parents contribute to these teenagers' comfort by providing everything they need, transporting them everywhere until they learn to drive, and providing a vehicle once they are driving alone. Today's teen generally has every material item any human being could desire and really can't understand why anyone would be in a hurry to move from this blissful state.

By actively decreasing your teen's creature comforts, you will help her quickly come to understand the value of a dollar and begin thinking how she will make her own way in the world. The following steps can be used to help your teen develop drive through the experiences of discomfort:

- Refrain from purchasing everything your teenager desires, such as cosmetics, decorative items, special shampoos, and so on. Just stick to the necessities.

- Do not provide a cell phone for your teen. If you truly believe she needs it for safety purposes, consider a service that allows you to completely control whom she calls and when she uses the phone, and monitor her minutes. There are great services today that will give you the control you need. If your child wants the comfort of what has become a teen pacifier, she will have to earn it through working. Teens can babysit, cut grass, help with household chores, and do many other things to earn money. Allow her the discomfort of being the only one without the phone to propel her into working for it.

- Require your teen to transport herself whenever safely possible. She should walk, ride her bike, or take public transportation at every opportunity. Don't hop in the car every time she wants to go somewhere. If you are concerned about safety and don't want her to have a cell phone, get a pair of walkie-talkies so you can communicate with her as she travels short distances. Encourage her to get her friends to come along so she has company.

- Refrain from providing continual entertainment for her in the form of television, computers, and so forth. Require times when she will need to read or make her own fun.

- Talk to her about life after high school. Be sure she understands your expectations. Tell her that you expect her to go away to a four-year college. Do not allow her to think staying home is even an option. Start preparing her by having her take on more responsibilities at home. Make it a little less comfortable for her to live with you each year so she can't wait to go! By senior year, she will have one foot out the door, as it should be.

- Most important, make sure your teen understands that she owns nothing. Everything that is in your home belongs to you. She has only the *privilege* of using the things as you see fit, as she earns them. Help her make the connection between creature comforts and having the money to afford them. Talk about careers that may be of interest so she starts thinking in that direction.

The Slow-Track College Student

Bill is twenty-three years old and is still in college. When his parents question him about how many credits he has or how long it will take to finish, he tells them to back off and avoids the issue. Bill bounces back and forth from apartments near campus and his parents' house, which is about a forty-five-minute commute. Sometimes he stays on campus for weeks at a time, and sometimes he stays home. His parents are never really sure if he will be home and kind of wait to see what will happen. Bill seems content with this lifestyle. He goes to lots of parties and has a perpetual string of short-term girlfriends. Though he's chosen a major, he really doesn't have any particular goal and doesn't seem to want to finish school.

Bill works about twenty-five to thirty hours a week in a video store. He is a good worker but never seems to have enough money to make ends meet. His parents pay for his car and give him cash to help with his food or rent when he is living near campus. They want to encourage him to stay in school, but they feel they are walking that fine line between being supportive and butting in, so they don't ask too many questions for fear that Bill might completely drop out.

Many college students move on a very slow track. Only slightly over half (52 percent) of students enrolled full-time in four-year institutions have earned their bachelor's degree in *six* years.* Average time of completion ranges between four and a half and five years. After six years, 14 percent are still enrolled and a whopping 32 percent have left college without a degree. Although students are not completing their studies, they are usually quite comfortable. Many take only the minimum courses required to retain full-time status. This can be as little as three courses per term. Many of them work in menial jobs to make enough money to maintain their vehicles, party, and entertain themselves. In a word, they become quite comfortable with the status quo. They are having a good time and see no need to hurry things along. The danger is that as each year passes, they are less likely to complete college or to find a true purpose in life. If you don't increase the discomfort at this stage, your children will end up moving back home with you and will have a whole new set of problems (see the next section). Here are the steps you need to take as a parent to prevent or interrupt this slow-track trend:

- Get your child into a four-year university setting as quickly as possible. If your child is not quite ready academically, encourage him to enroll in a community college with the goal of

---

* U.S. General Accountability Office, *College Completion* (Washington, DC: U.S. General Accountability Office, 2003), 11.

transferring to a four-year college as soon as possible. Students who spend two full years, or longer, living at home and attending community college are much less likely to earn a bachelor's degree.* The same holds true for students who transfer to a different school. Try to help your child stay at one institution the entire four years.

- Be sure your child is taking a full academic load, designed to be completed in four years. Although you want him in a four-year institution, you don't want college to take more than four years unless he is in a longer program as part of an academic requirement (i.e., a five-year bachelor's/master's combination). Many times counselors will advise students to take it easy the first couple of semesters. They often recommend fewer classes than necessary to finish on time. Generally, a student should be enrolled in about fifteen credits (five courses) per semester to complete the program in four years. Again, the comfort of less academic stress actually harms the student. The more courses your child gets exposed to early on, the more he will learn and the more he will move forward. College students often begin to explore different fields of study and then stumble onto something that fascinates them. If their workload is too low, they tend to get bored, work more, party more, and lose their focus.

  College should be about the academic work. While this may feel a bit uncomfortable at first, a student can usually learn quickly how to effectively manage his time and achieve success. While you don't want to be a helicopter parent and interfere with your child's counselor, be sure your child understands that *you* expect a full academic load. Most colleges have online systems that will allow you to check that your child is enrolled in enough courses.

* U.S. General Accountability Office, *College Completion*, 14.

- If your child is living at college, do not give him a car. I repeat: do not allow your child to have a vehicle. Though I encourage you to have your high school child drive himself where he needs to go when he's home, transportation can become a different story in college. Most college campuses are set up with transportation systems or are small enough that students can walk everywhere. Having a car on campus, however, can easily make your child very, very comfortable. He can go wherever he wants whenever he wants. He can come home and visit too often and go to too many places that distract him from his studies. He works more hours and is less able to take on coursework. Once students have vehicles, leaving campus tends to become their focus.

- Do not require your child to work very much during his college years. His focus should be on his studies as much as possible. Students who work more than twenty hours a week are less likely to graduate.* Students who really do need to work should consider federally subsidized work-study positions. These jobs are on campus and are worked around the student's class schedule. The numbers of work hours are limited, and workplaces are conveniently located. This is a great way for students to earn money toward their education without the stress that accompanies outside employment. Find a way through government assistance and loans to get your child's education paid for without undue hardship on him.

- Encourage your child to stay away from you, particularly in the first semester. Many students are very uncomfortable during what is usually their first extended time away from home. They get extremely homesick and tend to want to come home frequently, at every opportunity. The closer the college is to

* U.S. General Accountability Office, *College Completion*, 13.

your house, the more likely you will see your child every weekend. The more the student comes home, the less he will get
involved with college life. He will count on you too much and
will miss the many opportunities to gain the independence
he needs at this age. Talk to him about his feelings of homesickness and strategies to deal with these feelings, but require
him to stay on campus for at least four or five weeks at a time
without coming home. His discomfort will propel him into
activities and friendships that he might otherwise avoid.

- Encourage your child to get involved in college clubs or activities. Students who are involved in at least one activity are one
and a half times more likely to graduate.* Get on the school's
Web site so you can learn what might be available. Talk to your
child about what you think may be of interest. You may need
to make this a requirement freshman year to get him started.

The Parasitic Adult

Jennifer is twenty-five years old and lives at home with her parents.
She used to go to college but found it too stressful and boring. She
didn't have any particular career goal and didn't really see the point
of it all, so she left after a semester and a half and returned to her
safe bedroom in her parents' house. She waits tables part-time,
working three or four nights a week, and then goes out with friends
after work. She generally rolls back home around three or four in
the morning. Sometimes a few friends will come home with her and
have a late-night snack. Their favorite things to eat are sandwiches
and chips, usually cleaning out the fridge while they joke and laugh,
eventually waking Jennifer's parents.

Jennifer sleeps until noon or later and then moves slowly from
her bed to the couch, where she watches *A Dating Story, What Not*

* U.S. General Accountability Office, *College Completion*, 16.

to Wear, or any other reality show that TLC has to offer. She eats several bowls of cereal while she does this and doesn't concern herself with replacing the milk when it runs out. By the time her mom gets home from work at about five, she usually finds her way to the shower and eventually gets dressed. Her mom walks in the door and sees the remnants of this lifestyle and scurries to clean everything up before Jennifer's dad gets home. If he comes home and finds a mess, there will be a fight, and Jennifer's mom just wants to keep the peace.

Sometimes Jennifer joins her parents for dinner, and sometimes not. When she does, she gets grilled about what she is doing to better herself and who her friends are. Jennifer always retorts with statements about how she is an adult and how her parents shouldn't butt into her life and then storms off.

Jennifer's parents are at a loss. "We do everything for her," they say. They provide a vehicle for her to get to work, food, clothing, shelter, and lots of advice about what to do with her future. They are willing to pay for her to return to college. They encourage her, reminding her about how bright and talented she is, and urge her to go to college or find a more challenging job. Her mom takes care of the house and makes sure Jennifer's laundry is always done so that she will have clean uniforms for work. Jennifer's parents try not to cross the line, as they understand she is an adult and needs to make her own decisions.

But what can her parents do? "We can't kick her out. She is our daughter, after all," they say. They are completely perplexed. Jennifer doesn't seem to want anything and isn't motivated to change.

Jennifer's parents need to understand that they hold all the power in this situation. They own everything that Jennifer needs to live her life and have allowed her to live with them out of sheer love. Many parents believe they can't do anything. Yet they buy their children cars, clothing, food, and they let their children live without any responsibilities.

Jennifer's parents must create the need for their daughter to move by causing discomfort. They can do this in a series of steps so she will have a chance to adjust and make the necessary changes. Here is a list of possible changes that will create the drive that has been missing in Jennifer and perhaps your own adult child:

- Start with a very tough conversation with your child. Tell her that she has become too dependent on you and is not truly contributing to the family. Tell her that because you love her, you want her to have her own life and that you are going to take some very hard steps to point her in that direction.

- Require her to make payments to you for her vehicle and assume all responsibilities for maintenance and repair, and be sure she is paying her share of the insurance. If she cannot or will not make the payments, take the car from her. If you are worried that she will sneak out and drive it, sell it. Getting around without a car is very uncomfortable, so this is a great place to start!

- Stop doing her laundry or any other things that she can do for herself. She will do her own when she experiences the discomfort of having only dirty clothes.

- If she is the one home during the day, expect more from her. She should cook meals for the family, do yard work, or accomplish anything else that contributes to the well-being of the family. Make her understand that if she is living at home and is not contributing financially, her job is to be the family homemaker. Little by little, put more and more responsibilities on her until she feels uncomfortable with the job that has been thrust on her. If she happens to like this kind of work, you have discovered a career goal! Help her investigate opportunities in domestic service.

- Set very clear rules about guests in the house. If she comes in with friends who eat all your food, stop buying the things they like. Keep all meats frozen, and store snacks and cereals in a locked box out of the kitchen. If you don't want her friends in your home at all, firmly ask them to leave as soon as they attempt to enter. Take a stand on this. You are not running a restaurant or hotel!

- Take away her cell phone and any other communication device (including computers) if you are paying for them. Allow her to use the house phone or your cell phone to accept calls from potential employers or to arrange rides.

- If she is content sitting around and watching TV, lock the television in a cabinet, or use a child-proofing electronic device to block the signal during the day. This is similar to baby-proofing a house to prevent her from doing self-destructive things. Boredom is extremely uncomfortable. Eventually your child will want to do something and will get moving.

- Continue removing items of comfort until she desires to get them back. This will eventually create the drive she needs to move toward a positive future. Once she begins expressing this desire, you can provide advice and assistance to look for work or engage in meaningful education.

- Require her to pay rent. You should expect about 30 percent of her salary or fair market value for a studio apartment in your area. Make the rent high enough so that living with you will be no more comfortable financially than living on her own.

- If she does not make the changes you expect, you will need to kick her out of the house. Give her a deadline, and then stick to it. As an adult, she is not entitled to anything from you. She deserves an independent future, and you deserve to live your own life.

Children of modern America have grown up in an abundant society, with all the creature comforts a person could want. As they grow, they don't seem to want anything or desire to create a life of their own. Parents must help them connect creature comforts with drive and independence. If you continue to provide all the comforts of home, your children will never want to leave. To propel their lives forward, adolescents and young adults must feel the discomfort caused when these things are not handed to them. The desire for comfort drives people to work harder and choose professions that are more fulfilling. A person who wants for nothing has no drive, but material comforts are powerful tools that all parents can control and can use to increase drive.

EIGHT

6. Delay Gratification

Resist the Quick Fixes of the Lottery, Game Shows, and Reality TV

Have you seen the contestants on *American Idol* who cry after their initial audition when they are not chosen? Often they will say, "This was my only shot at making it as a singer!" They assume that everyone who is successful in the business has had a big break and fail to realize that making it in the music industry requires lots of hard work and perseverance.

Extreme Makeover: Home Edition is another perfect example of this phenomenon. The producers search for families who are down and out and make all their dreams come true. The more desperate the family, the bigger the payoff. While it is wonderful for these families, who are clearly in need, to have their lives altered so dramatically, it sends a terrible message: the recipients are viewed as highly deserving and entitled due to their misfortune; viewers often assume that the family would have been completely helpless to improve their own circumstances without the assistance of Ty, the show's host, and company. Young people who see this message over and over again on reality shows make the assumption that they, too, are entitled and deserving. They often just wait for someone to give them things instead of understanding their own power to make things happen.

If you listen for this message, you will hear it many times. You have probably even unwittingly delivered this message to your child. Did you ever see a really beautiful home or boat or other object you liked and say, "Well, when we win the lottery, maybe we can get that!"? I have caught myself saying that more than once, not really thinking about the message I was sending to my children. If your child hears that message repeatedly, she really will make the assumption that the way to material goods is through the lottery. She will understand that she cannot attain these wonderful things unless she wins them. In other words, she is helpless to alter her financial status except through some type of lucky windfall.

People who believe they are helpless to change their situation do not have any motivation to work to make things change. They don't seem to do the little things each day, or even to see the little things, that will help them achieve their desired goal. Many people play the lottery each day believing it's the answer to their prayers. Yet lottery winners often end up losing it all very quickly, ending up exactly where they were—or worse—before the big payoff. Reality TV and lotteries have created a sense of entitlement and helplessness in our culture, removing people's expectation of working hard to make their lives better.

What is a goal? According to Merriam-Webster's Collegiate Dictionary, it is "the end toward which effort is directed." Many people, however, tend to confuse a goal with a desire: something that hoped for. If a child asks for a bike for his birthday, it is a desire. But if he decides he wants a bike and devises a plan to earn the money for the bike, it becomes a goal. As a parent, your job is to help your child turn his desires into goals.

Waiting Is the Hardest Part

The point of delaying gratification is to teach a young person how to connect a goal with current behaviors. Someone who wants As on his report card will study every day. A person who wants to lose weight will eat less and exercise more. While these connections seem very simple, many young people fail to understand them. Children are inundated daily with images of people getting things just because they want them. A student can purchase test answers and papers online. Overweight people can have surgery and instantly begin to lose weight. Parents must aggressively teach their children how to wait for what they want and earn it through hard work.

I Want to Be Famous!

If you talk to the average adolescent, you will likely hear her talk about becoming famous. Young people today seem to equate fame with happiness and crave to learn about others who have already obtained fame. Their idols include people like Paris Hilton—famous for being famous—and many with quite questionable talent. Technology and a shift in our cultural appetite for reality television have made fame seem highly attainable. Anyone can put up a Web site or video for all the world to watch, and there are numerous stories on the news about people who have achieved fame through one of these processes. However, the grand majority of average Americans will never become famous. And that's not a bad thing.

This desire to become famous, and the belief that it is relatively easy to achieve, causes many young people to have false expectations about the realities of success and wealth. To combat aspects of this issue, try to prevent idol worship in your home. When I was growing up, my mom never allowed my sisters and me to put up posters of famous musicians or actors in our rooms. When I asked why, she told me that she did not want me to elevate these ordinary people to a status greater than the people in my own life. I didn't quite under-stand it at the time but kept that thought in my head throughout adolescence. When others were drooling over stars, I understood they were just people. Help your children understand that fame does not mean a person is any more important than other people. Instead, encourage your kids to go after goals that reflect true accomplish-ments—this is what will build feelings of self-worth.

Instant America

There is nothing slow about American culture. We use drive-throughs for coffee, dinner, lunch, breakfast, dry cleaning, prescrip-tions, groceries, and banking, which allows us to barely slow down on errand runs. Thanks to prepaid passes, we can speed through tollgates and pay without slowing down at all. We eat on the run, talk on the run, and put on our makeup on the run. Much of American business takes place in minivans, cars, and SUVs while parents drive their children from school to soccer practice. We get our news in sound bites, around the clock, and have an endless sup-ply of updates via computers that can be accessed anywhere at any time. Everything can be delivered to us when and where we want it. Technology can be carried to any location.

Although this fast pace allows us to get things done quickly and provides a great deal of convenience, it has robbed our children of patience and perseverance. Parents must reframe this context for their children to develop the work ethic necessary to sustain success in life.

Visualizing Goals

The movie, book, and related products known as *The Secret* have become runaway best sellers, promising purchasers great wealth and success just by thinking it will happen. Much of *The Secret* is actually repackaged parts of *The Power of Positive Thinking*, made famous by

Norman Vincent Peale. The basic premise is that you will attract the things you think about. If you believe that good things will happen to you, they will. Conversely, if you are in constant fear of doom, doom will find you. Most people would agree that a positive outlook on life is fundamental to happiness, fulfillment, and moving forward. Generally, when you emit positive energy, you will get more back in return. Try this simple test: if you see someone who looks down, smile at the person and say something nice. Almost always, you will get a smile in return, even from the grumpiest soul.

However, *The Secret* seems to dwell on material goods, causing some viewers to misinterpret the message. In one segment of the movie, a young boy imagines a bike. Almost immediately, the bike simply appears. The truth is that visualizing as is described in the movie and book *is* an important step in attaining one's desires, but one must usually be willing to make continual steps toward the desire for it to materialize. A parent can use the ideas of the law of attraction captured in the movie and book and expand on them to help a young person reach her goals by using the following eight steps:

1. Visualize the desire. If your child wants a new MP3 player, go to the store with her, and find the one she really wants. Get a picture or brochure with a picture of it. Or you might want to photograph her holding the one in the store.

2. Talk about the item and why she wants it. Discuss how she will feel when she uses it, the type of music she will load on it, and when she will listen to it.

3. Post the photos in her room so she will have a constant visual reminder of her goal.

4. Tell her to close her eyes and imagine using the device. Have her think about how wonderful it will feel to have it and imagine she is using it right now. Tell her to visualize in this way several times a day.

5. Come up with a plan for her to earn the money for the device.

6. Every day, ask her what she has done to work toward her goal. Discuss other ways she can earn money to reach her goal sooner. Keep asking, "What else can you do?" Get her in the habit of asking herself what else she can do each day to move closer toward that goal.

7. In the event she gets frustrated, whiny, or demanding about getting the device, remind her to close her eyes and visualize how great it feels (in the present tense) to have this item. Don't allow her to get stuck on ideas such as "I will never earn enough money."

8. As soon as she has raised enough money, help her make the purchase immediately.

This technique can be used for any goal, big or small. The bigger the challenge, the more important it will be for your child to visualize it and then work like crazy to make it happen. There are just three things your child really needs to remember: to visualize the end (in the present tense), to work hard, and to always ask herself, "What else can I do today to move closer to my goal?" Apply these steps to the situations detailed next to help your child learn to set goals and move toward them.

Middle School: Short-Term Goals

Middle school is a good time to teach your child how to reach the short-term goal of obtaining an item she desires. Every middle schooler wants a cell phone, and most are given the status symbol with no questions asked by the time they are ten or eleven years old. Parents have come to believe that the cell phone is a safety essential that must be in their child's pocket before she leaves the house. The truth is that most middle schoolers rely on the cell phone to talk to friends, text-message, and play games.

Parents can use this device as a way to teach delayed gratification. Instead of simply handing your child a phone, devise a plan for her to earn one and wait. This can be done by having her do extra chores or finding a way to earn real cash through delivering newspapers, assisting neighbors with yard care or child care, and so forth. The key is having her wait to get this thing by earning the money to pay for it. After your child has secured the actual device, she must continue to pay for it in the same manner. A cell phone is a great tool to teach this principle due to its relative inexpensiveness. Family plans allow you to add a line for about ten dollars a month, and the phone itself can be purchased for very little money.

High School: Long-Term Goals

Now that your child knows how to earn money to purchase something of value, you can move on to more long-term goals. High school students tend to start panicking because they don't know what they want to do with the rest of their lives. Our society has set the expectation that teens should know this. Middle schoolers and younger children can usually rattle off several things. As children develop a better understanding about careers, however, they realize that they don't really know what they want to do. Further, they think that selecting a college or choosing not to go to college is directly related to their career choice. We need to get out of the habit of treating college as job training. With a few exceptions—for professions such as teaching or engineering—college is not really designed to be job training. It is designed to produce well-educated adults. It is time to teach our children that we expect them to become well-educated adults. That is why we expect them to go to college.

Set the expectations of higher education early and often. Most students will have the opportunity to go to college. The question is what type of college they will have access to. If you want your child to strive to be the best student he can be, take him to see several colleges and universities. Walk through the campuses, and talk about what it takes to be accepted into the school of his dreams. Tell your child that you expect him to leave home after high school and to go to a great school where he can learn and grow. Talk through the kinds of study habits he will need to develop to make this dream a reality.

My son, although quite intelligent, was an average student. It was difficult to motivate him to get good grades because he really didn't see the value in them. He did, however, care about movies. He was so excited in middle school when a new Blockbuster store opened up a couple of miles away from our house. We got him his own card, and he started riding his bike there to rent movies. This created a wonderful sense of independence for him and fueled his love of the movies. Our dinner conversations turned into film-study classes. My husband would talk with my son about all the nuances of each film, comparing and contrasting the works of various directors, writers, and performers. By the end of middle school, Daniel wanted to be a filmmaker. But he still did not care at all about his grades. I couldn't figure out how to get him motivated until I stumbled on a solution almost by accident.

During Daniel's freshman year in high school, I had to take a business trip to Tallahassee and took him with me. We went on a campus tour at Florida State University (FSU). FSU has a wonderful film school, and we were able to tour that as part of our visit. Daniel was thrilled. He could not stop talking about FSU for the entire four-hour trip home. He started telling me how important his high school grades were and that he needed to earn mostly As to be eligible for enrollment at FSU. This one trip sustained Daniel's motivation all the way through high school. He made the connection between a goal and current behavior.

As it turned out, he was accepted into the university, but not the film school. In the end, however, that didn't matter. He ended up getting a dual degree in English and theater and following his love of theater upon graduation. It doesn't matter if your child knows what he wants to do for a living. As long as he is moving, he will get someplace. Just keep your child propelling forward.

If your child is interested in *American Idol*, learn the back stories of the contestants. The truth is that most of them have been working toward this goal for years. They didn't just wake up one morning and start to sing on TV. The show can serve as a good example of opportunity meeting preparedness. One has to be ready to take advantage of an opportunity by having the required skills in place. Assist your child in learning the truth about people who become "overnight successes."

Whose Money Is It?

As the old adage says, money isn't everything. The truth is that there are good people and bad people within every socioeconomic group. There are happy people and sad people within every socioeconomic group. There is no shame in having wealth and no shame in not having it. The important thing is to decide what kind of life you want to lead and what kind of messages you want to give your children about money.

Every child must be directly taught the value of a dollar. As children become older, they tend to demand more expensive things. They want the latest fashions, the best electronics, and any material goods that are popular at the moment. Oh—and they want it now! It seems that the more you give them, the more they want and the faster they want it. If you happen to have adequate means to provide these things, you probably take great pride in passing this wealth on to your children. But they need to understand one thing: although *you* may be incredibly wealthy, they have nothing. Really—they have nothing. Legally, they don't even own the toys in their room or books on their shelves. (The only exceptions to this are children who earn a lot of money through acting or some other professional pursuit. These children are protected by the courts so that their parents cannot squander all their earnings.) But basically, children are not adults and cannot own property.

Your children need to understand that they have only what you have given to them. It is critical to establish this distinction, particularly if you are a family of great means. By establishing your child's poverty, you establish your child's need to earn a living. This provides an excellent context in which to teach the value of a dollar and the process of delaying gratification.

Here are the steps to follow to teach this valuable skill:

- Don't give your child everything she wants. Children have a habit of asking for things constantly. If you normally buy whatever they desire, they will want for nothing and have no reason to work for things.

- When your child asks for something, ask her some questions about the item. Let's say it is a large-ticket item, such as a gaming system. Ask her how much it costs, how often she thinks she will use it, why she wants it, and so on. Help her determine just how badly she wants it.

- Be sure to distinguish between wants and needs. Many children will say things like, "I really need this." Ask her what will happen if she does not get the gaming system. Will she become ill? Will she die? Will there be dire consequences? Of course not. Most of the time, children want things that they have seen advertised or that their friends have. Be sure your child understands the difference between wants and needs.

- Once you have established the item's value to her, discuss ways that she might earn the money to get it. Does she have a job? Is she capable of getting a job? Are there other ways for her to earn money, such as babysitting, cutting grass, doing odd jobs for people in your neighborhood? Help her develop a plan for earning money to purchase this item.

- If it is a very expensive item that is clearly out of her reach, you may want to offer some assistance. For example, you can match every dollar she earns with a dollar that will become a birthday or holiday gift. You can also teach her to pool money that she may receive from other family members for a birthday or holidays.

- Establish a budget for your child's needs. Think about typical conversations when children and parents shop together for clothing. You can hear the same conversation over and over again. The child wants a pair of sneakers that cost over a hundred dollars, and the parent tries to convince her to go for the cheaper pair. The child tells the parent that she will be totally humiliated if she has to buy the cheaper ones. The parent, not wanting her child to be the only one in the Wal-Mart specials, finally relents and buys the more expensive pair. The shopping trip ends up double or even triple the original price. Instead of shopping for items and negotiating over what you will pay, put this burden on your child. This is also very helpful for teens who want certain shampoos and other cosmetics.

  - First, determine how much money you spend on your child's clothing, toiletries, school supplies, entertainment, and other items for the entire year. Leave school trips and special events out of the budget for now, as you will need to determine permission for these individually as they occur. Discuss this with your child so she understands just how much money you spend on her.

  - Divide the annual amount by twelve to determine a monthly budget for your child. Put this amount into your monthly budget.

- Sit down with your child, and share your monthly budget with her. Show her how much you spend on the mortgage, utilities, and other household needs. Help her understand where all the money goes and how you determined how much she will receive from you.

- Give your child her monthly allowance at a set time each month. Be sure she understands exactly what she must pay for out of this amount.

- Allow your child to make decisions for spending this money. You should still reserve veto power for clothing—but only for style choices. If she wants to blow her entire allowance on one outfit, that is completely her decision.

- Here is the most important part of this process—*do not bail her out*! Let her decide how to spend the money. She will probably make some mistakes. She may spend all her money on an outfit and then not have enough money to go to the movies with her friends. This will be very painful to watch, but don't bail her out. The only way your child will appreciate the value of a dollar is to be without enough money when she really wants something.

My husband and I put this process in place with our children when they were in middle school. It was amazing how quickly their behavior changed and how our conversations changed when we went shopping. Instead of arguing over the importance of name brands, my children began searching the sale racks and telling me how they did not really need a particular item. This was only possible after they lacked the funds to do something they really wanted to do. I felt myself aching for them, wanting to help, but resisted the urge. After a while, my children determined that their monthly allowance was not quite enough to do all the things they wanted to do. They started looking for ways to earn money in the neighborhood and were able to get odd jobs.

The key to making this all work is to set the allowance rate to provide for basic necessities and just a little fun. Then children learn the difference between wants and needs and seek a bit more. This practice will assist them in avoiding the credit traps that many young adults experience and will allow them to successfully manage money for life.

Children need to see the connection between goals, perseverance, and achievement. You must teach them this vital connection. Teach them the difference between a desire and a goal. Teach them to visualize their goals and continually keep their goals in sight. Teach them to take every step imaginable every day to move closer to the goal. Most important, teach them that they are capable of achieving and deserving of that achievement through hard work.

7. Encourage Accomplishment
Create a Sense of Self through True Achievement

The students are lined up ready to march when they hear "Pomp and Circumstance." They look so formal in their caps and gowns and seem to stand a little taller. It's hard to believe that four years have gone by since the more playful days of their childhood. Parents look on, so proud of their children's accomplishments. The future looks so bright for these students! Tears flow as each student receives a diploma and a congratulatory handshake. Photos and videos are taken continuously throughout the ceremony. Afterward, caps are tossed into the air. Graduates pose with proud parents. Students receive cards and gifts, and the families go off to restaurants and parties with their highly educated children, who have achieved so much in their young lives.

It is wonderful to praise these graduates. They certainly must feel proud of themselves. They know they are entitled to the accolades bestowed on them. They are worthy, high achievers who have worked so hard and sacrificed so much to reach this momentous milestone, right? Well, it would be if these were college graduates—or even high school graduates. But they are preschool graduates. They are four or five years old and experiencing what is the beginning of a lifelong phenomenon of modern American culture that rewards nonachievement rather than real accomplishments.

Look on the applications of many community sports teams, and you will find that your participation fee includes a trophy. It seems that somewhere along the line, we decided that every child gets a trophy! During the self-esteem movement of the 1980s and 1990s, that seemed like a perfectly good idea. It was thought that competition was bad and that rewarding each person, just for coming to the game, was good. Certainly, there could be nothing wrong with giving each child a tangible acknowledgement of his or her participation?

Consider this example: Susie joins the recreation soccer league at the age of seven. She shows up for most of the games. Sometimes her team wins, and sometimes they lose. Sometimes they don't keep track of points because it is just about having fun. Susie enjoys being on the soccer team, meets some new friends, and develops some new skills. At the end of the season, the entire team goes to the local pizza joint and has a party. The coach hands Susie a trophy and tells her that she, along with all her teammates, is a winner! Susie would have been perfectly content having fun, meeting new friends, and developing some new skills. But now she learns that she is so talented at soccer that she gets a trophy! Pretty cool, right?

Wrong. Susie does not understand what she has done to earn this trophy. Being with new friends and mastering new skills are their own reward. Susie's self-esteem grew by doing that. She didn't need to get a trophy and to be called a winner. When everyone gets a trophy, nobody understands what it takes to strive and move forward. A child gets the idea that there is a prize for showing up.

Employers have noticed for the past ten years or so what problems this practice has caused. Employees sometimes believe they should be rewarded simply because they come to work. Many employees have little or no concept of the connection between quality work and raises or promotions. A childhood full of unearned trophies leads to an adulthood of feeling denied by not getting undeserved rewards.

What Really Builds Self-Esteem?

During the 1980s, there was a great deal of research on self-esteem. Self-esteem was defined as feeling good about oneself and thinking one is smart, funny, nice, and so on. There was much media hype about the link between high self-esteem and achieving athletic success, choosing not to do drugs, earning good grades and income, and every other indicator of a happy, successful life. It was the magic potion to a wonderful future for every child. As a result, school districts, youth organizations, and families demanded that every child-serving organization assist children in developing this trait.

Textbook companies, toy companies, and educational suppliers rushed to develop games, programs, books, and paraphernalia to enhance self-esteem in children and adults. Educators were trained to give every child a prize when playing games in the classroom. Sports leagues began rewarding each participant with a trophy. Many schools had complete programs on self-esteem, helping children declare, "I am somebody." They engaged in daily cheers and chants, developed rituals about feeling good, and focused on this important issue.

Children who were being raised during the 1980s and 1990s understood they were wonderful, beautiful, brilliant, and artistic—even if they weren't. The result of all these efforts is what we are seeing now: a generation of young people who think they are entitled to receive all the world has to give without really working for it. We need to move toward rewarding accomplishment to instill real self-esteem and drive into this generation.

By the end of the 1990s, we began to learn that it is not the amount of self-esteem but a realistic sense of self that is the most important. Although the research at this time was extremely clear, it went virtually unnoticed. It is natural for parents to want their children to feel good. We love going to preschool graduations and sports banquets to watch our children get trophies. Parents crave the feel-good moments that these types of events produce, so they orchestrate even more of them. Competition is stressful and sure does not feel good if you are on the losing end of it. So many parents strive to eliminate competition from their children's lives.

Once, when interviewing a potential student for my school, I fielded an unusual question. I was explaining that we have spelling bees each quarter to encourage children to become better spellers. The seventh-grade student I was interviewing asked, "Does everyone get a ribbon or trophy for the spelling bees?" When I explained this was not the case, that only the winner received a prize, the student turned to his mother and told her that he did not want to attend our school. When I attempted to explain to the parent how healthy this type of competition could be, it fell on deaf ears. The mom did not want her little darling to be subjected to losing, so she was off to find a school that would always tell her just how wonderful her son was.

Why Is Competition Important?

Healthy competition is critical in developing drive. Think of a communist country in which all workers are treated exactly the same, no matter how hard they work or how much they produce. They all get the same pay, according to the government's wage scale. They all live pretty much the same way. In a capitalist society, it is different—hard work and production are rewarded, and those who do a better job get the spoils. Of course, even a meritocracy is not a perfect system. There is a great deal of inequity. People in very important jobs, such as teaching, are not rewarded as much as those in other careers, such as sales. Sometimes bosses are biased toward certain employees. The alternative, however, is that nobody ever gets ahead because everyone is the same. It is critical that we raise our children in a way that prepares them to participate successfully in a capitalist society.

No parent wants to see his or her children lose. It hurts too much to watch your child suffer. So we often want to construct our children's lives in a way that reduces this pain by reducing competition. But losing and failing from time to time are what teach us the most important lessons. Think about a turning point in your life when you suddenly knew what you were supposed to be doing. Think of the times when you learned the most. Chances are that your epiphany was related to a failure or loss. Failure, and all the pain it brings, is the fuel that inspires us to achieve and leads us to all that is truly important. What we often forget is that children need to experience losing to desire winning. As a parent, it is your obligation to allow your child to experience failure and all that it brings—and then to help him deal with it. Use such experiences to teach life's important lessons. Only then will you prepare your child for the realities of life.

The Desire to Win

This desire to win is at the heart of drive. Isn't it a good thing to want to be the best at something, whatever it may be? Instead of shielding your kids from competition, focus on identifying healthy competitive experiences for them to participate in. Establish a culture of healthy competition within your family that will allow your children to still feel good after an experience that does not result in winning. You can have board game competitions, running and swimming races, kickball games, or any other fun event that will teach kids how to win and lose gracefully. When your child loses, be sure to congratulate her for the things she did well. Point out her successes, and help her understand what she can do to improve.

Creating a healthy competitive environment in your family
- Don't let your child win at card or board games. Play the game with integrity.
- Teach your child as you are playing so that she will benefit from your experience and get better at the game. Once she is competent at the game, slowly remove the assistance.
- If your child loses a game, talk with her about what she did well. Ask her what she could do next time to improve her chances.
- Be sure your child understands that losing at a game does not translate into being a loser.
- When your child wins, congratulate her for a job well done, and ask her what she thinks you could have done to improve your chances.
- Be sure she understands that winning a game doesn't mean she is better than the person who lost. You want her to be a graceful loser and a humble winner!
- Talk about how much fun you had playing with her and how you look forward to a rematch so she will have a chance to beat you—or you will have a chance to beat her!
- Find a sport or outdoor activity that you and your child can become skilled at together. This could be riding bicycles, skiing, playing tennis, fishing, or anything else you can enjoy together. Learn about equipment, take lessons, and enjoy each other through this activity. It will provide wonderful moments of playful competition that will be loads of fun for you both!

- Always encourage your child in any competition. Encourage effort and improvement. Never berate her or call her names when she strikes out or doesn't win.
- Be careful not to connect winning at sports or other activities with tangible rewards such as bikes and toys. Although it is great to celebrate a success, avoid prefacing a game with "If you win today, I will buy you a new toy."

One of the most important factors to consider when choosing competitive activities for your child is the demeanor of the person leading the activity. For example, a Little League coach who berates children when they strike out is not someone you want to work with your child.

There will probably come a time when you will encounter a coach or activity leader who treats your child unfairly or does something that has the potential to impact his self-esteem in a negative way. You will be tempted to allow your child to quit. Don't do that. Instead, help your child understand what the coach is trying to accomplish. Many times a child will say things like, "He keeps yelling at me. He is making fun of me." Find out exactly what the coach is saying. Kids often use the word *yelling* when they don't like what someone is saying. Most of the time, the person has not raised his voice and is providing important feedback to the child. Ask your child what the coach said exactly. Was the coach truly raising his voice or just being stern? Ask your child why he thinks the coach was saying those things and what he can learn from them. If, after your conversation, you are still concerned, go to the coach (without your child's knowledge), and see what he has to say. If you think he is truly trying to help, talk with your child and help him understand what the coach is trying to accomplish. If you think the coach is doing things that are harming your child, be very specific and tell him what he is doing or saying that you believe might be harmful. Then watch the coach in action and confirm what he is doing.

It is perfectly acceptable, and desirable, to have a coach who does not hesitate to point out your child's flaws and help him fix them. Even if your child finds that feedback embarrassing, explain to him that it will help him get better. Encourage your child to develop a tough skin that will enable him to use feedback to improve and to not take it as a personal attack.

It is acceptable in many instances for a coach to raise his voice on the field to make a point or get the team's attention. What is *not* acceptable is name-calling, berating, or screaming right in a child's face. Your job is to determine what the coach is doing and to address it if it is not acceptable. However, don't let your child quit the team unless the coach is being truly emotionally or physically abusive. If you let him quit midseason or midgame, you will teach him that when things get tough, you can just walk away instead of rising to the challenge.

The Real Goal

My son played soccer for several years. He was a wonderful team player, but not the most athletically inclined kid on the field. The coach was great; Daniel played in every game for at least a quarter and got to try almost every position. Thankfully, the coach was wise enough not to put Daniel in the goal box!

Daniel played with great spirit, pride, and courage. He couldn't wait to get out there at every opportunity and improve his game. The coach worked closely with him to teach him the finer points of the game that would help him improve. The coach was always encouraging and built up Daniel's confidence.

Daniel had been playing soccer for about three years. Although his team always had a good record, he had never scored a goal. His dad and I had never talked about this with him and hadn't really thought much about it, since he played defense almost as much as offense. Instead, we focused on specific things he did in each game that were positive and talked about how he could improve. Toward the end of the third season, somehow, miraculously, Daniel scored a goal. I can remember that moment as if it were yesterday. He had possession of the ball and moved toward the net. He used his left foot to angle the ball toward the center of the field and then made his move. For me, watching in the stands, everything seemed to move in slow motion as he hoisted the ball through the air, over the head of the goalie, and into the net. Everyone on the team and on the sidelines jumped in the air and screamed! Most knew Daniel for the entire time he had been playing and understood how much heart this kid had. They were as thrilled for him as my husband and I were.

At the end of the game, we packed up our things and started walking toward the car. Daniel looked at my husband and me and said, "I'm done now." When we asked what he meant, he told us that he wouldn't be playing soccer next season because he had scored a goal. Apparently, getting a goal had been his goal. Although he experienced the sheer joy of playing and had always been on a winning team, he had had a very personal—and very private—goal of scoring just one point for his team. Once he had accomplished that, he decided it was time to move on to other things. I was kind of stunned. Daniel had never told us about this desire. But somehow he was slowly driving toward that and felt so much accomplishment from achieving it that he no longer desired to play soccer. Instead, he wanted to move on to a new challenge.

It is important to understand and encourage your child's individual goals within a sport or other competitive activity. Remember to focus on what *he* wants to achieve. Don't assume that winning or getting to a certain level is what he wants. It turned out that my son did not care at all about winning. We discovered that his only desire, outside of just having fun with his friends, was to score a point. After that season ended, Daniel never played soccer again. He turned his attention to other sports and always quietly set his own personal goals for achievement. This practice has spilled over into all areas of Daniel's life and allowed him to always keep his goals in sight and within reach.

Many of us can be tempted to relive our own childhood moments through our children. If some type of success eluded us, we somehow think we can re-create the possibility of achieving it through our kids. This is the most dangerous type of parenting! It robs children of their own identity and makes them believe they are nothing unless they reach *your* goals for them.

There was a young boy named Scott on Daniel's soccer team. This kid was absolutely gifted. As Daniel was working for three years just to score one goal, Scott was leaping and dancing across the field with absolute grace, scoring at least half of the goals at each game. He was elegant in his athleticism and certainly appeared destined for greatness in the sport. Daniel and Scott were friends and seemed to appreciate each other, despite the great chasm between their ability levels. Scott's dad went to every game and paced up and down the sideline so that he would always be as close to his son as possible when Scott was playing, which was most of every game, in the center-forward position.

Toward the end of the second season, Scott's dad thought that his son was beginning to slack. So he devised a reward system to motivate Scott. For every goal, Scott would get ten dollars. If the team won, Scott's dad promised him a bonus. When Scott missed an attempted goal or made some terrible error, his dad would take away a dollar. As Scott moved up and down the field, his dad would grandly announce his total for the game. Every single time Scott made contact with the ball, his dad would let the world know how much money he had just earned or lost.

This went on for several games as we watched all the joy disappear from Scott's face. His elegance turned to robotic movements. His smile faded and his eyes seemed to sag. At one point, Scott sat down on the field. For a moment, we thought he was hurt but then understood he was drained from the pressure. His father screamed at him and called him horrible names. Scott stood up, with tears in his eyes and a defeated expression on his face, and tried to play once more. He made contact with the ball and heard his finances being broadcast for the last time. He looked over at his dad; dropped his head, shoulders, and heart; and walked off the field away from his dad. He just kept quietly walking toward the parking lot as his father followed, still screaming. A brilliant career crushed by age twelve.

Of course, this is an extreme example of a parent putting ridiculous pressure on his child to win. But think about how you or other parents you know approach competition. If you provide tangible rewards for winning or forget why your child is playing, you will diminish the wonderful benefits that healthy competition can provide.

The opposite extreme of Scott's dad is the parent who won't let a child compete at all. There are many parents who will only let their children play sports when no score is kept. These parents shield their children from competition at every turn, convinced it will somehow destroy their children's very fragile self-esteem.

Competitive Advice, Age by Age

OK—so you have made the decision to teach your child through competition. How do you do this in a world that attempts to insulate young people from failure? You first need to make the decision not to participate in the everyone-gets-a-trophy culture. Then seek out opportunities for your child to compete in ways that are healthy and promote growth.

Middle School

Middle school is a time when children should be trying everything so they can develop joys and passions in life. Here's some advice on teaching your middle schooler through competition:

- Expect your child to continually try new things, and discuss the joys and difficulties in doing so. Allow her to express her fears if she is worried. Be sure that at least one of the chosen activities includes competition. Do not expect your child to identify the activities on her own. If she is not sure what she would like to do, provide her with two or three possibilities for sports and the same for the arts. Allow her to choose the one that is most interesting to her.

- There may come a time during this new activity that your child wants to quit. She may perceive that she is being mistreated or tell you that participating in the activity is uncomfortable. Do not give in; be sure to investigate the issue. Unless your child is being physically abused or harmed, require her to finish the activity.

- If your child doesn't get the part she wants in the play or the position she wants on the team, help her learn why. Encourage her to talk with the leader of the group about this issue. Do *not* do this for her, no matter how upset you become when she is overlooked. Have her ask the question exactly like this: "Can you tell me what I can do differently next time to get that part/position?" This is the only appropriate way to approach a coach or director. At home, help your child understand this information. Be careful not to attack the coach or director. Instead, assist your child in understanding how to get what she wants the next time.

- If your child's sports team wins, help her understand what they did well that caused the win and what things were pure luck.

Do the same when they lose. Discuss what they can do better the next time to increase their chances of success.

- Help your child process her feelings when she wins or loses. Help her learn from both experiences.
- Pay attention to the closing rituals of an activity, such as banquets and parties. Many sports subscribe to the everyone-gets-a-trophy philosophy, rewarding every player with trinkets just for participating. If this is the case, opt out of the closing event.

High School

High school is a time when young people may become extremely afraid of failure and, as a result, fail to try. To teach your high schooler not to fear losing or being picked last, consider these suggestions:

- Require your child to participate in at least one new school activity or organization each year. This can be a competitive sport, the school play, or an after-school club. Require him to participate fully by going to all practices, rehearsals, and meetings.
- Talk about the organization's successes and failures and what caused them. If your child is not selected for something he wants, help him understand what caused this to happen. Encourage him to go to the leader of the organization and ask, "What can I do differently next time to get the part I wanted?" Avoid blaming the leader of the organization. Instead, help your child understand how to do better with this person next time.
- Require your child to work or volunteer each year. This can be for a limited time during the summer or for short hours during the school year. Help him prepare for required interviews by putting together a résumé and practicing the interview process. If he is rejected, discuss his feelings with him and brainstorm how he can do better the next time.

- For each activity, discuss with him what the leader or boss will expect. Ask him what a good team member/cast member/employee/volunteer should do. Make a list of attributes of a person in this position, and assist him in developing these attributes in himself.
- Every step of the way, talk about successes and failures and what can be learned from each. Assist your child in processing his feelings and helping him understand that he is still the same person regardless.

Young Adults

Young adulthood should be a time of great opportunity and exploration. Talk with your child about her immediate and future goals. Be careful to stay away from questions like "What do you want to do with the rest of your life?" It is very unusual for someone just out of high school to know that. It can be quite difficult for the young person who doesn't go to college to find her way. To assist her in developing a sense of self and purpose during this difficult time, follow this advice:

- Discuss what she wants from life right now. Does she want to move out of the house? Take some classes? Travel?
- Where does she see herself in four or five years? Where does she want to be living? What kind of car does she want to drive? If she has difficulty identifying these things, take her to visit places and test-drive cars to gain some perspective.
- Once she has developed a vision for her future, you can discuss what it will take to get there and the competition that she will be fighting to achieve her goals.

Vocational school/job training. For some young adults, vocational school or job training, which prepares students for a specific job or career, is the best option. Such programs can sometimes be very competitive, with high-paying jobs on the line. You can assist your child in gaining a competitive edge with the following advice:

- *Every moment in class is a job interview.* The person teaching the class is usually a working professional or someone who has much experience and many connections in the field. Every teacher can bring you closer to securing a job in the future. Treat each day in class as a job interview. Dress appropriately, arrive on time, be prepared, and behave yourself.

- *Prepare well for each class.* Only those who are ready to engage in learning will be able to take full advantage of each learning opportunity.

- *Visit possible job locations in your community.* Tell them you are a student and want to learn more about the field. Most professionals are eager to share their experiences and can provide great connections for the future.

- *Talk with the job placement service at your school early and often.* The better the people there know you and like you, the more apt they will be to help you get a job.

- *Be nice to everyone.* You never know who will be your connection to a good job.

College. The purpose of a typical liberal arts college is to provide an education that will give your child multiple perspectives on the world. A college graduate should be a well-educated human being. The purpose of a typical liberal arts college is *not* to provide specific vocational training. Even students enrolled in specific professional preparation programs, such as teaching or nursing, must fulfill the liberal arts education requirements if they are enrolled in a bachelor's degree program. It is critical that you, the parent, understand the purpose of a college education. Students will often say, "I don't know why I am taking this class—I will never use it." If you are sending your child to a four-year institution with the purpose of pursuing a bachelor's degree, you are paying that institution to educate your child in the broadest sense of the word. The focus of these four years should be intellectual, cultural, and social growth. Your child should emerge from the college experience more aware, insightful, and intelligent.

This time of life can be very frustrating for a young adult, particularly if he is not yet sure what he wants to do after college. There is a great deal of pressure for him to make up his mind. Relax. Many of us are still trying to figure out what we want to do well into middle age. Most of us will change careers completely at some point. Some of us may change our minds two or even three times. Life is an exciting journey full of possibilities. Help your college student understand there is time to figure out the far future. While he is still in college, assist him by advising him to do the following:

- *Take classes in subjects that are interesting—for any reason.* A bachelor's degree typically includes many elective credits. This is intended to provide the student with an opportunity for exploration. Many people find their passion in life by accident when they take elective classes. A student can also parlay elective credits into a double major, giving him a competitive edge later on.
- *Work hard and get good grades.* Although learning should always be the goal, college grades are often critical in the highly competitive world of grad school admissions and in job interviews. There will be times when your child experiences an unfair teacher or a subject that holds no real interest for him. Tell your child that you understand this, and help him to find the areas of study he *is* interested in and to achieve the grade he needs. Teach your college child to ask each professor his or her criteria for achieving in the class. Each professor should provide a syllabus at the beginning of the term detailing how the grade for the class will be determined. Talk with your child about this important document. What will he need to do to get an A or B?

- *Don't cheat.* Emphasize to your child that cheating in any form is never acceptable. There is a pervasive cheating culture on many college campuses. Many students believe there is nothing wrong with copying material off the Internet or peeking at an "advance copy" of the test that someone has pilfered. But there is: not only is cheating morally and ethically wrong; it can result in dire consequences. Students who are caught can be expelled. Those who do elude being caught will usually not do as well overall as students who earn their grades fairly. Eventually, robbing yourself of a good education will catch up to you. Many high-achieving students are tempted to help others cheat to earn money. Talk to your child about better ways to make money. Help him understand that he is diminishing his own competitive edge by selling his work to others.
- *Take advantage of every opportunity presented, and find new ones.* If your child is interested in anything, help him find out how to pursue it.

Alternatives to the Everyone-Gets-a-Trophy Culture

You can make a decision not to participate in the everybody-gets-a-trophy culture. Choose not to attend the trophy ceremonies at the end of each sports season. Choose a preschool that doesn't "graduate" its students, or just don't go to the ceremony. Talk to your child's teachers about how they provide tangible rewards. Get involved and talk with other parents about how to counteract this trend. Be sure that you are aware of the culture in your own home. Be careful about what you reward and how you reward it. Instead of paying for good grades, consider celebrating an accomplishment as a family by going out to dinner together. Talk to your child about balancing effort and success, and help him make the connection between the two. Praise him for working hard and truly accomplishing something that was difficult. Let him see you struggle to learn new things and talk about how gratifying it is. If you get a raise, promotion, or award, discuss what you earned and how you earned it.

A child also needs to know that hard work is its own reward. Cleaning out the garage or weeding the garden shouldn't always translate into dollars. Work with your child at home or in the community for the joy of contributing without expecting anything in return. Self-esteem comes from working hard and succeeding, not from getting a trophy every time you show up.

Key concepts of healthy competition
- Children should receive tangible rewards only when they truly earn them, not just for showing up.
- Children need opportunities to see work as its own reward.
- Children need to make the connection between effort and success; help them understand that by sharing your own work and rewards with them.

Self-esteem is developed through true accomplishment. And true accomplishment is only possible when your child is allowed to take risks. Competition is a part of life. If you don't allow your child to experience it, he will be ill prepared to participate in a full life. Think about the things your child will need to do as an adult—being accepted into college, getting a job, securing a promotion, and achieving excellence in the arts or sports all involve competition. It is your job to help your child understand how competition works and how he can be successful in a competitive world. While doing so, you must continue to encourage him by helping him understand that losing experiences have a silver lining. He can often learn the most from his failures—including what it will take to succeed the next time—and can gain valuable life experience from enduring them.

8. Control the Crowd
Use Peers for Positive Influence and Independence

Erika's mom, Lynn, was awakened at about one in the morning by a frantic phone call. It was Erika calling from the local police station. Erika had been driving friends home and was stopped at a checkpoint set up to snag drunk drivers. Although her blood alcohol level was slightly below the legal limit, Erika was only sixteen and was therefore charged with underage drinking. There were three other teens in the car who were also charged. Lynn quickly threw on her clothes and raced to the police station to retrieve her daughter.

When Lynn arrived at the police station, she found her daughter in tears. Erika was so distraught that Lynn began to feel that this was punishment enough. She couldn't imagine how traumatic it must have been for Erika, being put in handcuffs and hauled to jail as if she were a serious criminal. "Kids make mistakes," said Lynn. "I'm sure she learned her lesson." When Erika explained that she had "only a little" to drink and that her highly intoxicated friends had pressured her into driving them home, Lynn really understood.

She had been worried about these friends for a while. Lynn knew her daughter was a good girl and had just fallen in with a bad crowd.

Thankfully, Erika was eligible for a diversion program, allowing her to avoid more serious penalties. She would, however, lose her driver's license for six months and had to see a counselor every week. Lynn agreed with Erika that this seemed extreme and went with Erika to see the counselor and tried to have him reduce the suspension. Lynn explained that Erika needed her license to get to and from school and work. She also explained to him about the bad crowd and said that she would be sure Erika would no longer hang out with these kids. Erika felt relieved that her mom would help her in this situation and that her mom saw Erika wasn't at fault.

I wish I had a dollar for every time I heard a parent tell me, "He is not a bad kid. He just got in with a bad crowd." Who is the bad crowd? I very rarely hear a parent acknowledging that her child is completely responsible for his own behavior. Parents tend to blame those other kids who are influencing their own sweet, precious baby. Many children who have been in trouble will parrot this statement and truly believe that if it weren't for "those" kids, they would never have had a problem. Remember, other parents will be referring to your child as one of "those" kids. If your child has behaved badly or exercised poor judgment, avoid using this excuse. In Lynn's case, she should have also focused on Erika's behavior—that she broke curfew, had been drinking alcohol underage, and then drove after drinking—and held Erika responsible for the consequences.

That said, the influence of friends certainly leads to many behaviors, good and bad. Children must be accountable for their own behavior, *including* the selection of their friends. To help your child have the greatest chance of success, you must teach her how to select successful friends and remove herself from them if they start making bad choices.

You need to help your child understand your expectations of his friends. Let your child know that you expect him to identify friends who have dreams and goals. Teach him to start looking for those qualities in others. If his current friends don't have those qualities, help your child find ways to widen his circle of friends until it includes others with goals and dreams. You do this by requiring him to participate in new activities and to go to new places where he will meet other young people who can be a better influence on him.

A good, positive, driven friend will:

- Want to try new things and encourage your child to do the same
- Want to stay out of trouble and encourage your child to do the same
- Care about learning and schoolwork and encourage your child to do the same
- Think about the future and encourage your child to do the same
- Be kind to others and inclusive of other friends

You set the criteria, and your child is accountable for producing a peer group that meets your expectations. While it is true that you can't completely choose her friends, you can influence her choices by controlling communication and access to her friends. If at any point you believe a particular child is harming your child, you need to tell your child that this child is no longer a part of her world. Your response should be "I am the parent, and it is my job to help you surround yourself with people who will be a positive influence on you. This person does not meet my criteria, and you will not hang out with her." Now, we all know that you cannot control your child's relationships while she is in school. You can, however, control whom she sees and communicates with outside school. Deny her access to this person. Keep reiterating the issues, explaining that you do this out of love and caring. Help her understand that you want to be sure she runs with the good crowd. Vetting your child's friends needs to include how those friends behave, what those friends' goals are, and how those friends treat your child. Adolescents develop relationship skills that determine their future marriages, work relationships, and so on. Your job is to assist your child to demand the treatment she deserves from others.

How do you know if your child's friends will provide the influence to help him become driven? Unfortunately, young people tend to drift toward mediocrity. To understand this phenomenon, one only needs to understand very basic physics, like Newton's first law of motion: an object at rest tends to stay at rest, and an object in motion tends to stay in motion with the same speed and in the same direction unless acted upon by an unbalanced force.

Once young people get themselves into a safe circle of friends, they tend to want to stay with that group rather than venture out into the world. You will see them going to college together—or staying home together. They will just want to be together. Doing so feels good and safe. But the danger is that they stay at rest and choose not to broaden their horizons. So take a look at your child's friends, and determine how driven they are. The more driven the friends are, the more driven your child will be.

Who Are Your Child's Friends?

If you want your child to be driven, you must assist him in selecting friends who demonstrate that they are motivated. A teen or young adult can be derailed very quickly when surrounded by others who are only interested in hanging out or cruising the mall. A group of friends will normally sink to the lowest common denominator; the one negative person can pull every other member of the group down with him. Your job as a pathfinder parent is to assess the drive of every child who influences your child and to encourage your child to select friends who are driven. The tough part of this job is to discourage relationships or sometimes even force the end of a relationship that is robbing your child of drive.

At this point, you are probably wondering how in the world you can actually manage your child's friendships. Many parents will say things like, "I can't choose his friends for him." While that is true to a certain extent, you can and must assist your child in evaluating friends and their impact on his life. This is a process, not a single decision on your part. Parents who are effective in this area talk continually with their child about each friendship. They help him recognize and appreciate the traits of drive in others and to develop it in himself.

You absolutely can influence your middle-school-age child's friendships. Talk about the important qualities a friend should have, and help your child identify those qualities in others. Every time your child establishes a new friendship, invite that child to your home and talk to him over a pizza. If that child is obviously not the type of friend you want for your child, make it clear to your child that his contact with that person will be severely limited.

Of course, the younger the child is, the more control you have. However, you can control many things even with a young adult. You need to understand the power you have—both tangible and intangible—to influence this. One of the positive qualities of Generation Me is that they value their parents' opinions and want to be close with their parents. Use this to your advantage whenever you are concerned about your child. Don't be afraid to get involved and tell your child what you think about his choice of friends.

To form an opinion of your child's friends, you will need to learn a lot about them by talking with them and asking them key questions. My daughter, Alison, used to get very upset when I would "interrogate" her friends in this manner. I explained to her that as a parent, I needed to get to know her friends. I told her that these were people who were important to her, so they were important to me. She told me many times that I made her friends nervous with this line of questioning. Now, those few who were truly bothered by it didn't come around much. Most of her friends, however, seemed to enjoy the attention (teens love to talk about themselves), and the questions got us into some nice conversations about life and their futures and helped us get to know each other well.

If one of her friends seemed to completely lack drive, I would point that out to Alison. I would ask her what she thought that person would be doing after high school. We talked frequently about the importance of spending time with other people who shared high expectations for their futures. I wanted her to know that if she was connected to people who were satisfied with mediocrity, then she would feel bad striving for more. Exposing hopes and dreams to others who have none makes one the object of intense suspicion and ridicule. Therefore, it is critical to find like-minded souls who share a desire for greatness, or at least an expectation for an interesting life.

How to Get to Know Your Child's Friends

To get your child's friends to open up to you, it is important to make them want to spend time in your home and feel comfortable when they are there. Assist your child in arranging gatherings and fun activities that will attract others to your home. This might be a gaming system, a pool, a pool table, or just pizza. The point here is to be the place where everyone wants to hang out. You will never get to know your child's friends if they are always someplace else.

Once you are successful in drawing his friends to your home, do all you can to make them feel welcome. Introduce yourself and take an interest in them, just as you would any guest in your home.

Many parents make the mistake of getting out of the way as soon as their child's friends arrive. At some point, of course, you will want to make yourself scarce. You should, however, plan on spending a little time with your child's guests first.

Be sure you have lots of food on hand, and assist your child in serving it. Sit down and share a slice of pizza or some cookies still warm from the oven. This is the very best time to conduct your questioning.

Later, after the friends have gone home, you can discuss their responses with your child. Really help your child understand whether his friends are driven and why you believe that. Reiterate your expectation that he surround himself with driven friends and why it is important.

Drive Questions

The following lists are questions you can ask your child's friends, based on their age.

Middle school students

- *What do you like to do for fun? What are your interests?* The child should be able to discuss something other than hanging out, playing video games, being on the computer, or going to the mall.
- *How is school? What is your favorite subject? What do you like about that subject?* The child should be able to speak about something he or she enjoys at school (other than lunch and recess) or a favorite teacher.
- *What are your dreams for the future?* Many children don't really know what they want to be when they grow up, and that is really OK. What you are looking for here are dreams. These could be about traveling, a type of home or car, or other things the child would like to experience.

- *Do you do things to earn money?* Many children are simply given everything they want. You are looking for responses that indicate a child is expected, and wants, to earn things.
- *What do you think you will do after high school?* Kids with drive will have some ideas. They usually want to leave home. They may want to go to college or tech school. They may talk about staying home and working to save up and leave home. You are looking for some thoughts about the future.

High school students

For high school students, ask the same questions listed for middle school students plus the following:

- *What do you plan on doing after high school?* If the child talks about college, ask what college or type of college (big, small, nearby, or faraway). If the child says, "I don't know; I guess I will just hang around here, maybe go to community college," the child is inert. If the child talks about something other than college, look for specifics—like the type of job or the technical school he is interested in.
- *How are you preparing for that?* Once you have identified what the child is planning after high school, ask things that tell you that the child knows what it will take to get there and is working toward that goal. The child should be able to tell you very specifically what the requirements are and what he is doing to accomplish those things he specified.
- *Where do you stand in the high school completion process? How many credits does it take to graduate from your school? How many have you earned so far? How are your grades?* Many high school students (and their parents) have very little understanding about what is required for high school graduation. Driven teens continually evaluate where they are in the process and make adjustments to reach their goals.

- *What are you doing this summer?* Summer should be a time for relaxation. It should also, however, include something of interest. Again, you are looking for some plans. Kids without drive tend to hang out at the mall, sleep in, and so forth. Those with drive will talk about doing things. This might just be a little bit of travel. The key is that they are actually thinking about doing something.

Young adults, post high school

The term *post high school* describes any young person who is no longer in high school. Remember, almost 30 percent of young people don't finish high school, so chances are that one or more of your child's friends will be in this category. You do not want your child hanging out with others who have not finished high school and are inert, even if—especially if—your child is one of the 30 percent. A young person who has not finished high school needs to be surrounded by others who will help him move past what has caused this problem. Questions to ask your child's young adult friend include:

- *What are you doing these days? Are you going to school? How many credits are you taking? Are you working? If so, how many hours? Are you doing other things?* Try and determine how much of his time is accounted for in structured activities. If you don't hear enough things that add up to full-time school, full-time work, or about forty hours a week, that is a red flag.
- *Tell me about work (or school)? What do you find interesting about it? What are your interests?* He should have some interests beyond video games, going out partying, or hanging out at the mall. Driven people are continually finding new ways to learn, grow, and have fun. You are looking for curiosity and excitement about life.

- *What are your goals for the future?* Possible responses include a job, where he wants to live, aspirations, dreams, and so on. You are listening for indicators that he is moving. Remember the law of motion: an object at rest tends to stay at rest, and an object in motion tends to stay in motion with the same speed and in the same direction unless acted upon by an unbalanced force. You need to determine whether your child's friends are at rest or in motion.

My children used to refer to this line of questioning as "the interrogation." But it really wasn't that bad. It was just a conversation that we would have over a meal in the kitchen. The result? Often that the child who was the "victim" of my interrogation would return, asking for help working toward these goals. By taking an interest in a child, you actually help him. He will know that you are open to conversations about his future. You may be the only one in his life to take an interest, so don't ever be afraid to be interested.

An Unbalanced Force

So what if your child is headed in the wrong direction or is at rest? You need an unbalanced force to interrupt her life and push her in the right direction.

My daughter, Alison, is very driven. She had always wanted to be a singer and did everything in her power to pursue this goal—until her junior year of high school. Tragically, one of her friends died that year, creating an unbalanced force that interrupted her forward motion. Understandably, she suddenly became very connected to her other friends. They formed a little cocoon around themselves. While this was completely reasonable in light of what had happened, and even desirable for a short period of time, eventually her father and I became concerned about how this was going to affect her future. It seemed as though Alison had begun to lose her sense of purpose, resting instead of moving.

Alison was headed toward her senior year and needed to prepare for her auditions for music conservatories. These auditions are extremely competitive, and it seemed her voice was suffering because of her grief. Much of what had interested Alison in the past suddenly did not interest her anymore. Her friends were all planning on staying local or going to the same state college together after high school, and she was interested in doing the same. My husband and I were not quite sure what to do. We have always believed that just because you can doesn't mean you should. Someone who is musically talented should not necessarily pursue a career in music. Alison was blessed with an amazing voice, but if she chose to do something else with her life, that would have been fine as well. We had never really pushed her into music but always ensured she got what she needed if she chose this for her career.

As her junior year came to a close, we felt it was critical that she make a commitment to voice if that was what she chose. Yet it seemed increasingly more difficult for her to focus because she was so caught up in being with her friends. Alison was in constant fear that she would lose someone else, and she seemed to want to hold on tight. So we gave her a very strong ultimatum. We told her that we would support whatever she wanted to do. If she wanted to focus on her friends and take things slowly, going to a local college, that would be fine. If she wanted to audition for conservatories, that would be fine, too. However, if she chose the conservatory route, she was going to commit 100 percent. We told her that we would only pay for her auditions (which included a great deal of travel and expense) if she left her high school. She would have to finish her remaining credits through an online program so she would be free to focus on the music. She would have to spend less time with her friends and focus only on herself and her future so she would be fully prepared for conservatory auditions and ultimately have the musical preparation necessary for success at the college level. We created an extreme force in her life to unbalance her and make her choose a direction. This is the only way to combat the inertia that is inherent with becoming entrenched with a group of friends.

Alison chose, after much anguish, to leave her high school and focus on her music during senior year. At the time, she thought we were being extreme. However, as she went to her auditions, she thanked us for forcing this issue. She ended up getting accepted at two of her top choices of schools. Without taking this step, Alison would not have been able to pursue her goals.

If your child's attachment with a group of inert friends is stalling him, try the following strategies:

- Travel. Go on an extended trip with your child. If you travel with your job, consider taking him with you on some trips. Expose him to lots of different cultures, perspectives, and ideas.
- Send your child away to a camp or precollege program for an extended period. This will encourage him to forge new friendships with other driven young people and to create a new circle of friends.
- Take your child to visit a college or school that would be interesting to him. Talk about the kinds of students who go there and what it will take to get in.
- Require your child to try an activity or sport that is new to him so that he will experience a new circle of friends.
- Continually evaluate and discuss the level of drive among his friends, and help him identify the kinds of people who can help him grow as a person.
- Talk to your friends to help find other young people who might have similar interests. Don't be afraid to "fix up" your child with new friends.

Being a Parent, Not a Friend

Some families face the opposite problem. Kaitlyn, for example, doesn't have a close group of friends. She would rather be with her mom. "My mom is definitely my best friend," she says. It is with her mom that she shares clothes and shoes, gossips about boys, goes shopping, and does pretty much everything. Kaitlyn would prefer to be with her mom than anyone else, and Kaitlyn's mom wouldn't have it any other way. "I think it's great that my daughter feels this way about me—after all, we only have each other," her mom says. Kaitlyn's dad has never really been in her life, so her mother feels fortunate that she has a daughter to be close to and spend time with.

A normal part of an adolescent's development is to begin separating from parents and other family members. A preteen or teenager wants to develop his own unique identity. He wants to be more independent and begin to create his own life. This is a very healthy process that normally begins during the middle school years. During high school, it becomes even more pronounced, with the teenager feeling closer to some of his friends than his own family members. Eventually, a young adult will move out of the family home. Only then will he really understand his relationship with his family and begin to develop a mature, close relationship that will support him emotionally as he lives his own life. This is how it is supposed to be. I've seen many parents struggle to understand why friends had become so important and why family had become somewhat less important during this time but then become gratified when their child moved back toward them emotionally as he started life on his own.

However, many of today's young people have stopped following this very normal, very healthy developmental path. Instead of moving away from the family, they are now clinging tighter to their parents. It is not unusual to hear a teen proclaim that his parents are his best friends, that he depends on them for emotional support, that they do everything together. Teens spend much more time with their families than ever before, at the expense of developing normal, healthy relationships with their peers. Of course, these parents are delighted! They had always heard of all the teenage angst and feel so fortunate that they are not experiencing this. They are thrilled that their children would prefer to live at home than in a dorm during college. Everything is great—until they realize their twenty-three-year-old has taken up residence on their couch. Then they start to get concerned. Is this kid ever going to leave home? Will I ever be able to make a study out of his bedroom? Will he ever get married and have a family of his own?

Remember, you are the parent. You are not your child's friend. Maybe someday, when he is a completely independent adult, you can be. But even then he will still need your guidance and your unedited advice about mistakes he is about to make or just made. You can and should enjoy spending time with your child. You can share similar interests and have great conversations. But if your child is relying on you for all his social interactions, you have a big problem. When a teen proclaims that his parents are his best friends, this usually makes the parents feel all warm and toasty inside. However, you need to get past this and allow your child to get his own friends. A friend cannot discipline his friend. A friend cannot make the hard choices and steer the child in the correct direction. You are a parent and will always be a parent to your child.

What are the warning signs of parent-child friendships? You might be more of a friend than parent to your child if:

- Your child says you are his best friend.
- Your child frequently turns down invitations to be with his peers to spend time with you.
- Your child talks to you about gossip around school as if you were his buddy.

- You worry that your child might get mad at you when you discipline him. You may find yourself apologizing for disciplining or saying something like, "We're still friends, right?"
- You regularly find yourself saying things like, "I like you—you are my friend."
- Your child often joins you when you go out with your friends.

There are two reasons that parents may subconsciously encourage their children to cling to them and not to develop their own friendships. First, the parent needs friends herself and has come to rely on the child to fulfill her own social needs. Second, the parent fears too much that the child will get caught up in the wrong crowd and be influenced in a negative way by friends.

OK—you have created too friendly of a relationship with your child. How do you turn that around and begin to be the parent? Consider the following measures:

- When you are disciplining your child, stop worrying about your child's anger. Chances are he *will* be angry when you discipline him. This is usually affirmation that you are making the right decision.
- Get your own friends. Be sure you have a couple of people you enjoy spending time with to avoid the trap of relying on your child's company for your own social fulfillment. This is especially true for single parents.
- Once in a while, kick your child out of the nest. If you see an opportunity for a positive social experience—like a school dance, a party, or other teen event—insist that your child attend. You may have to actually require this. After the event, help him process the social interactions that occurred and his feelings. Teens will naturally feel left out at times and might question whether they belong. This is completely normal and part of the developmental process. Help him understand that

everyone his age feels this way, and teach him how to work through it.

- If your child is having difficulty connecting with his current peer group, help him find new places to develop friendships. Consider clubs and organizations, youth groups at places of worship, community theaters, and so on. You can help him develop interests, and then he will gravitate toward other young people with similar interests.

- Have small gatherings at your home so he can pick the people he wants there. Remember, your job is to supervise, not to be a guest.

- If your child is still having difficulty, find a camp or other overnight experience that will force him to have sustained involvement with a peer group away from you. You may have to force the issue and tell him that you expect him to do this.

Every child needs a good core group of friends who will encourage, push, and challenge him. Your job is to teach him the value of good friends, to show him how to select the friends who will move him toward his goals, and to shake things up if he needs a new direction. Only then will your child have the drive he needs to move forward.

9. Create a Sense of Purpose
Make Life Meaningful

Brianna is twenty-five years old. She has a decent job in an office that provides enough money to pay her bills. After graduating from college at the age of twenty-three, she lived with her parents for a while until she could get a job that paid enough for her to live independently. She has a little apartment where she lives with her cat. Every day she goes to work and performs the tasks she has been assigned. She goes out occasionally with friends and has a good time. Brianna enjoys swimming and reading and seems to be well adjusted.

But one day when she went to work, she pulled into her normal parking spot and just sat there. She could not bring herself to go inside. She felt paralyzed, fearing that something terrible would happen to her if she set foot in that office even one more day. For about twenty minutes, she held on to the steering wheel, staring straight ahead, sweating and breathing heavily. Not knowing what else to do, she picked up her cell phone and called her mom. She could not describe this feeling but was only able to tell her mom that she was coming home. On the way to her parents' house, she realized what the problem was. This new job was not fulfilling to her. She knew that it was not for her and that she needed to do something else. She had no idea what, but she knew she needed to make a change. Brianna ended up quitting her job and moving back in with her parents, who were completely stunned by this turn of events.

Brianna is not alone. Like other people her age, she is not driven by anything in particular. She is not sure what she wants or what her purpose is. She is not even sure how she is supposed to figure this out. Purpose creates intense drive. Knowing why you are here on earth ignites a fire that is difficult to extinguish.

Why am I here? What is the meaning of my life? At some point, you have probably asked these questions. Human beings have a natural curiosity and need to understand their purpose. In his landmark 1943 paper, "A Theory of Human Motivation," renowned psychologist Abraham Maslow proposed that each person has a set of basic needs. He arranged the five categories of basic needs in a pyramid. According to his theory, an individual must meet the physiological needs from the bottom before reaching the top group of needs that includes self-actualization. It is during the time of self-actualization that a person explores his purpose in life.

In many places in the world, a person may never reach this point because he is still concerned about survival. We, however, live in an affluent culture where our basic needs are usually met from the time we are small. The more affluent the home and community, the sooner a person will reach the point of needing to explore self-actualization.

People who lack purpose often finds themselves in crisis. We're all familiar with the example of a midlife crisis when a middle-aged man starts questioning all the choices he has made and suddenly develops a need to reexamine his life, sometimes acquiring a new sports car or girlfriend in the process. Suddenly, the person looks

Self-Actualization
Achieving individual potential

Esteem
Self-esteem and esteem from others

Belonging
Love, affection, being a part of groups

Safety
Shelter, removal from danger

Physiological
Health, food, sleep

Abraham Maslow's Pyramid of Basic Needs

around and says, "Is this it? Is this all I am supposed to do?" During this time, many people make major career changes and determine what their true priorities are.

But there is a new phenomenon in the United States that young people are experiencing called the "quarterlife crisis," which typically occurs during one's twenties. This is the time after college when the young person suddenly realizes that he has no idea where he should be going or what he should be doing. He may not be married and may still live in his parents' house. He just can't seem to find his direction or purpose. Parents of twentysomethings in the throes of this crisis kind of scratch their heads trying to understand how someone who has everything could be experiencing such angst. And therein lies the problem. This situation often comes about because the young adult has been provided with too much—too much food, material goods, shelter, safety, and comfort—which may cause a sense of entitlement. In other words, he already has everything included in Maslow's lower four categories of needs. Psychologically, he moves immediately into the top tier of the pyramid upon reaching adulthood, but he doesn't know what to do now that he's there.

Purpose

When we talk about finding our purpose in life, we are answering the most difficult of life's questions: "Why am I here?" Many middle-aged adults cannot answer that question, so you can imagine how daunting it may be for a teen or young adult. Parents with religious affiliations often immerse their children in faith, attempting to steer them toward an answer. Rick Warren's best-selling book *The Purpose-Driven Life* has helped countless people around the world discover what they consider God's purpose for their lives. Churches have adopted the strategies in Warren's book to help their parishioners understand God's purpose for them. While this approach may work for a few young people, it is certainly not right for all. Kids need to discover what is truly important to them. It could be a life serving God, or it could be skateboarding. It could be taking a stand against animal abuse, singing with a band, taking care of children, or writing. Finding one's purpose may be related to earning money, although it is not necessarily so. For the luckiest of us, our purpose opens a way to earning money. There are many people, however, who do one thing to earn money and find their purpose in volunteer work or hobbies.

Helping your child find purpose happens over time through many events and conversations. You have to watch carefully and truly pay attention to see what is important to your child. To help your child find purpose, it is important that you create an environment in which he will have a wide variety of experiences that allow him to find his place in the world. Every experience is an opportunity for you as a parent to help your child explore his values and priorities. The trick is in the processing. Following is a strategy that can be applied to many events and activities to assist your young person in understanding himself a little better. These suggestions will help him establish his values and see how they relate to his place in the world.

Try using this line of questioning after your child has completed an event or activity or started a new job or hobby:

- Tell me what you liked. If your child cannot pinpoint anything, prompt him: Was it the place where the activity took place? Was it the people? Was it the feeling you had while you were involved?

- Tell me what you didn't like. If your child cannot pinpoint anything, prompt him: Was it the place where the activity took place? Was it the people? Was it the feeling you had while you were involved?

- Have you experienced something similar that you liked/disliked?

- Is this something you think you would like to do again? If not, were there things you liked that you might want to experience in the context of another activity?

- Now we know that _____ [the things he liked] are really important to you. We should start looking for other opportunities to help you experience that again.

Rachel and Patty's Story

Rachel was really mad at her mom, Patty. Patty had arranged for her to visit a college campus the summer before her senior year in high school. She'd be going for two whole weeks to take part in the school's science program. But Rachel fought and fought so that she would not have to go. She couldn't imagine having to leave her friends right in the middle of summer to go and study. Why would her mom make her do that? But Patty did not give her any choice.

Patty was going away on a cruise, and Rachel was sure her mom was stashing her at this camp so she could go and have a good time.

After Rachel returned home, Patty asked Rachel what she liked about her experience. Rachel said, "Nothing. It was stupid." Patty probed a little more saying, "Oh, come on, Rachel. I know you had to like something about it. You are still in touch with some of the girls from the trip." Rachel explained that liking some of the girls had nothing to do with it. She told Patty that she hated science and was furious that she had to go; liking a couple of friends didn't change that.

Patty told Rachel that she completely understood Rachel's anger at being forced to do something but that she still wanted to hear more about the trip. Patty asked Rachel about the friends she had made while she was there. Patty asked her what she liked about them and if they were any different from her friends at home. After a little while, Rachel finally said that she thought they were a little different. She said that she loved her friends at home, but that these girls were a little more serious about school and actually seemed to want to learn things that Rachel thought were hard.

Patty kept talking to Rachel about this experience over the next couple of months. What they discovered together was that Rachel had not been pushing herself academically. She had been kind of coasting through school and attaching herself to friends who did the same thing. But at the college, it was different. Rachel felt a little more free to show how smart she was. She had liked being around all girls instead of mixed in with boys. She liked that the girls were from lots of different places around the country and that they really liked to learn. Rachel and her mom decided that she should look for a college where none of her friends from home would be attending. Rachel kept in touch with her new friends from the summer and started looking at colleges they were considering. She even began to consider an all-women's college.

Patty helped Rachel discover what was important to her. She gave her daughter a brand-new experience, very different from anything else Rachel had tried before. She insisted that Rachel go even though she was scared and didn't want to go. After Rachel came home, Patty did not accept Rachel's simple responses to her questions. She continued to ask her to identify things that she liked and disliked until Rachel figured out what she liked about her new friends. Rachel discovered that learning new, challenging things was important to her. She learned that she wanted friends who were academically motivated. She started thinking that an all-female environment might be more conducive to her learning. Rachel did not learn what she wanted to do to earn money, and she did not completely change as a result of her two weeks at the college summer program. But she did start to identify one of her values and find a group of friends that felt safe. This is a big step toward finding purpose.

Chuck and Vincent's Story

Chuck played baseball his whole life and loved the game. He was happiest when he was on the field, breathing in the smell of freshly cut grass and the leather of his glove. Although he was not quite good enough to play in the majors, he did enjoy a couple of seasons as a minor-league player.

Chuck works in the insurance industry, but he spends all his spare time on baseball. He volunteers as a coach, plays on a local adult league, and goes to just about every home game of his local pro team. When Chuck was in his late twenties, he and his wife had a baby boy named Vincent. Chuck was thrilled that he now had a son with whom he could share his love of the game. Even before Vincent could walk, Chuck was tossing a baby-size baseball to him to get him started. Vincent played T-ball at the age of three and started with the local peewee league when he was only six. Vincent was OK at baseball but didn't have the natural gift that

Chuck demonstrated at his age. Vincent seemed to love the game, too, but what he really loved was his dad's attention. Baseball was the thing they could share. It brought them close together in a way nothing else could. As Vincent grew, Chuck was certain that Vincent shared his purpose.

But one day, when Vincent was about thirteen, he informed his dad that he no longer wished to play baseball. He still wanted to go and watch the local pros play but did not really want to play himself. He was a teenager now and was getting interested in girls and music and other things. Playing baseball was extremely time consuming, and he wanted to have a chance to explore other interests.

Chuck was stunned and extremely worried. He feared that Vincent would kind of drift around, not able to find his way in the world. Chuck didn't understand that that is exactly what Vincent was doing. During his high school years, Vincent tried everything he could. He played in a band and began writing stories. He played several other sports and enjoyed just hanging out with his friends. Little by little, he cut back on the time he was spending with his dad and baseball and spent more time on other things.

By the time Vincent was ready to go to college, he was totally confused about what he wanted to do. Chuck was still worried because Vincent seemed directionless. He thought quitting baseball had been a terrible mistake for Vincent—at least if he had baseball, he would have something. So Chuck kept talking to Vincent about what was important in life and why he loved baseball so much. He talked about the camaraderie that made him feel like part of something bigger than himself. He talked about enjoying the outdoors. He talked about the work ethic and tenacity that it takes to improve. He talked about how the rules of the game gave it an important structure yet allowed for strategic thinking.

As Vincent began college, he realized that he did share his dad's values. He loved being part of a team and being outdoors. He enjoyed working hard and overcoming obstacles. He liked rules but was always engaged in strategic thinking. One day while walking across the college campus, Vincent noticed a display where an army recruiter was standing. On the display were photos of a group of soldiers in various situations. He stopped to talk with the recruiter and suddenly understood his own values and what he needed to do with them. The recruiter spoke of soldiers who worked as a team to overcome obstacles. When Vincent asked about specific jobs in the army, the recruiter told him about several choices that were outdoors. What Vincent really loved was the structure that encouraged strategic thinking. The army was definitely a place where he felt people shared his values and where he belonged. Vincent decided then and there to be a part of it.

Chuck had no idea that sharing baseball with his son would result in Vincent joining the army. He was just sharing his passion for the game. Without knowing it, Chuck had gone well beyond the game and shared his values with Vincent. He connected things about baseball to things that are important in life. Vincent shared his dad's values and found his purpose by finding a world that includes them. Someone who has found his purpose puts himself in a world where he can honor what is important to him every day. Values create purpose, and purpose fuels drive.

What Does Purpose Look Like?

Individuals who are confident in their purpose are highly motivated because they are driven by something bigger than themselves. These individuals have difficulty understanding why people want to retire because they find their work so fulfilling. They are generally satisfied most of the time, regardless of income or current circumstances. They understand that they are secure in their place in the world.

Spotting an adolescent or very young adult with purpose is not as easy. Purpose in a young person looks a little bit different. Except in rare cases, young people express a different sort of purpose. For them, it might be playing on a particular sports team or singing in a choir. They are driven by the sheer joy of participating in something they love. Sometimes they love an activity because all their friends are participating with them. Other times it is because they have a talent for it or think it is fun. Children focus on what feels good today. They want to enjoy the moment and soak it all in. Many adults have difficulty with this. Such parents continually badger their children to figure out what they want to do for the rest of their lives, focusing only on what they will do to earn a living. While it is fine to ask these natural questions, it is just as important to ask kids what they like to do for fun, what type of place they might want to live in after high school (city versus small town; warm versus cold; big college versus little college). Parents should talk to their kids about things they enjoy right now and what they value about those things. These conversations should be relevant to the child's present and help connect it to the future, instead of the other way around.

On the other hand, here is a teen without purpose: when you talk to this teen, he is usually pleasant enough and doesn't do things that rock the boat. He is unable to identify things he likes to do or anything that has much of any interest for him. There is no spark in his eyes, no passion, no real motivation to get off the couch. A teen without purpose has difficulty finishing school. He can't even see past next week, let alone next year. Therefore, he will not have the motivation to move forward with his life. This is the kind of young person who will generally live at home with his parents well into his twenties, thirties, and beyond. If you want to help a teen like this establish a life of his own, you must help him develop some interests and passions in life that will motivate him to want something away from the very safe, sheltered existence he is currently enjoying.

It is important to note that teens are usually not yet equipped to determine their ultimate purpose or career goals. However, the trend in education is to require them to do just that. Many schools are adopting an educational approach that stresses the new three Rs: rigor, relevance, and relationships. Most people understand rigor (the coursework needs to be challenging) and relationships (kids need teachers and other adults to connect with them in a meaningful way). Most people, however, misunderstand relevance. They usually equate it with job training, believing that students should begin career planning as early as middle school. Parents and teachers tend to think about relevance as preparation for a career in the future and making money. But teens cannot think that far down the road. Something is relevant for a teenager if it involves friends or interesting and fun activities. A child may not want to be a professional musician, but band is sometimes the only thing that is relevant in the child's high school life. Usually, the meaning of life for teenagers does not extend beyond their teenage years. Be sure that you remember what relevance means—and does not mean— for your teen.

Giving

Children who grow up in an affluent society, where things are generally provided for them, have difficulty understanding that the rest of the world may not be like that. One way people, young and old, can find purpose is by giving to others. This can be through many acts, both great and small, close to home or abroad. It can be a response to a crisis or the result of seeking out others in the community who may need assistance but do not know how to ask. Parents who volunteer and regularly give can help their children do the same. Through giving, many people discover what is really important to them. Here are some ways that you can help your child give back:

- Once or twice a year, work with your child to sort through clothing and personal belongings. Start with your own things so she will get the idea. Have her help you figure out which of your clothes you no longer need. Together fold them carefully, and pack them into boxes. Try not to use garbage bags because you want her to understand that the clothing is going to help other people, not go in the trash.

    As you are doing this, talk with her and help her understand that other people could really use these clothes. Try to avoid phrases like "poor people" or "those less fortunate." You want her to understand that people are people. You can follow the same process for books, household items, and so on.

    Next, tell her that it is her turn to sort through her clothing and personal belongings. Identify the things she no longer needs that can be given to other kids who could use them. Load everything in the car, and take it to a local thrift store, charity, or other location that accepts donations. Talk about how valuable these things might be to others, how much you have, and what you do to get material things. Remind your child of our responsibility to help others every day and what a privilege it is to be in a position to do so.

- Find a community service project to get involved with together. This might be something small, like a weekend cleanup of a park, or something big, like going on a trip to help rebuild homes for flood victims. The more self-absorbed your child has become, the bigger the project should be. This should be something you can both do together. You may need to insist that your child participate.

Identify several projects that you think will fit in with your schedule and other needs, and then let your child pick the project. Before you engage in this activity, talk about why it is important. Then talk about what you think might be fun about it. After you finish the project, debrief the same way Patty did when Rachel returned from her trip to the college program.

- Help your child find an organization in the community that regularly provides volunteer assistance to others. These opportunities might be school based, faith based, or community based. These types of organizations are usually a great place for your child to connect with friends as well.

- Help your child learn to give money to charitable organizations. If she earns an allowance from you, ask her how much she thinks she should donate to others. Investigate places that receive donations to determine the best places to direct your money.

- Consider gifts of charity for the holidays. Some families make donations in a family member's name to that person's favorite charity.

- Consider adopting a family in need for Thanksgiving, Christmas, or Hanukkah. Local charities can help you identify a family. You and your children can make it a holiday project to make that family's holiday as joyful as yours. If you can't find a family, look for "angel trees" at local malls or stores. These are usually trees that have ornaments with individual children's names and their holiday wishes listed. Your child can actually pick out a personal gift for the recipient. It makes the giving seem very real to even very young children.

- Most important, be a good role model for giving. Be sure that your child hears you talk about how important it is to give to others, and be sure your child is aware when you donate to charity or volunteer your services. Involve her in every way possible.

When we find our purpose, we are finding where we fit in the world. To do that, we must find things that are bigger than ourselves and get involved. Giving and volunteering are great ways to discover that.

Making Connections

Most kids connect very readily with other kids who are like them. If they like sports, they hang out with athletes. If they like theater, they hang out with theater kids. They generally make friends at school or other places they frequent. Their mobility is limited, so they naturally stick close to home. They also feel most comfortable with others who are the most like them. Kids will even start to dress alike, walk alike, and talk alike as they move toward adolescence. A child's true purpose in life, however, may be very different and/or distant from where he is now. To learn more about the world and all it has to offer, a child needs exposure to lots of different people.

Elliot grew up in a small southern town and went to the local public high school. Everyone at his school was into football and school dances and hanging out. Elliot participated in these activities and really liked his friends. But he always knew he was a little different. He was an artist who was constantly drawing and creating. He loved clothes, which was very unusual for a boy, particularly where he grew up. Elliot had no idea what he wanted to do with his life. He just went along every day, enjoying his fairly normal teenage existence. Mike, Elliot's dad, was an engineer and really didn't understand why Elliot spent so much time drawing and thinking about clothes. He was concerned about his son, who didn't seem to be capable of thinking beyond next week. Mike couldn't get Elliot to talk about his future, college, work, or anything. Elliot didn't talk with his dad about anything of importance. They got along fine, but it was always surface conversations about sports or school.

At Mike's office, there was a guy named Tom who also loved art. He was in charge of marketing for the company, and he was always talking about going to art shows. Tom was impeccably dressed every day and seemed to love all the same things that Elliot did. So one day, Mike talked to him about Elliot. Mike asked Tom to take Elliot to an art show and maybe talk with Elliot about his job. Elliot and Tom connected really well in a way that Elliot and Mike were not able to do. Tom didn't replace Mike; Tom just helped Mike reach his son on a different level. Sometimes kids won't listen to their parents about life's most important issues. All parents need others to help their child see things from other perspectives.

In my work as an educator, I have been a parental accomplice countless times. Parents will come to me and ask me to help them steer their child in a particular direction or connect the child to someone with comparable interests. A parent simply cannot be everything to a child. You need to reach out to others to help get your child connected to the bigger world. Find other caring adults (whom you trust will have no ulterior motives) who can help your child find his place in the world, and engage their help.

Spirituality

Finding the meaning of one's life can often be found through spirituality. This can take many forms that may or may not include organized religion. Generally, parents raise their children in their own religion. As kids grow up, they often take on their parents' beliefs. Once they reach adolescence, however, all bets are off. A child who is brought up in a strict religious home may rebel and completely distance himself from his family's beliefs. Another child, brought up in an atheist home, may suddenly discover God through friends, join an evangelical church, and attempt to convert his parents. A crucial part of parenting is assisting a child in developing a spiritual identity. This part of being human shapes how we see the world and influences how we interact with others around us. Spirituality moves people to do amazing things and keeps them from doing others. It is important that you determine how you will foster your child's understanding of spirituality as she is finding her place in the world.

If you are like most parents, you have shared your religious practices (or lack thereof) and/or rituals with your child. If you go to a church or temple, you have likely required your child to go with you and enrolled her in classes and activities where she learns about your religion. You may have also allowed your child to go to other places of worship with friends and family members so she could experience other denominations. These are all positive activities that can help teach a child about spirituality, but they don't always get to the heart of the matter. Kids are very curious about what their parents really believe. Have you had conversations about how you truly think and feel about matters of spirituality and their impact on your life? Have you discussed where you think we go after we die and what we are here for? It is perfectly OK if you haven't figured this all out yet; many adults haven't. But sharing your uncertainty is equally as important. If you are on a personal quest to discover your thoughts on spirituality, involve your child in the process. Likewise, if you are really sure of your beliefs, share them with your child. If you are unsure and worried about it at the moment, that is important to discuss as well. Encourage your child to talk with others about this issue, as appropriate. Help her process this critical issue of humanity.

If you are interested in having your child participate in youth groups or other faith-based activities, you will want to consider these activities the same way as all others. Think about who is running them, the safety involved, and how the activities will impact drive. Some parents have the misconception that everything that happens at a faith-based function is automatically safe and inherently good for their child. While this is most often the case, you need to be certain. And you should ensure that your child has a healthy balance of activities that doesn't rob her of time to just be a kid.

Culture

Where you spend your time will naturally influence your perspective on the world. Most of us spend most of our time in a very small place, seeing the same people and doing the same things every day. If you want your child to find her place in the world, you need to show her the world. Now, most of us don't have the time or resources to be world travelers, but you can accomplish much of the same thing without going very far. Think about where you live and what is nearby. Think about places that your circle of friends frequent and places that you have never been. This might be as simple as taking your child to a diner across town where a whole different group of people live. You might go to a different type of movie or concert than you normally would or attend a festival that attracts people different from you. When you do go on vacation, go to a place you've never been, or get off the typical tourist route and spend some time with the locals in a family-owned restaurant. You may want to consider allowing your child to go on educational trips that travel to cities or other countries.

After each of these experiences, talk to your child about cultural norms. This simply means how people behave and talk, how they do things. How do they interact with each other? How has their environment influenced them? What do they eat, and where do they spend their time? Help your child become a sort of anthropologist, examining what makes people do the things they do.

While actually going to different places is the best way to accomplish this, reading, television, and the Internet are also great ways to start conversations in this regard. Read books and magazines that expose you to lots of different cultures, and share your insights with your child. Watch television shows on National Geographic and other stations that explore the world. Get lost on the Internet learning about other people around the world. Most of all, provide a context for your child to understand why we do the things we do and why other people do the things they do. This will help her understand where she might want to live and work as she grows up.

If you have helped your child experience lots of different things, taught him to give, helped him explore the meaning of life, exposed him to a variety of venues, and connected him with a wide variety of people, chances are something has gained his attention. Keep talking about what is important to him. What does he value? Help him discover what is truly important to him. How and where does he want to live when he is an adult? Assist him in understanding how different venues and lifestyles will impact him. What steps will it take to get to that point? What kind of education? Think about skills and habits he will need to develop. Help him create a sense of purpose today that will propel him toward tomorrow.

The previous eight steps to drive have been setting you up for this last, most important step of finding purpose. Remember, someone with drive wants to do things and be things. He learns to overcome tremendous obstacles to achieve success. He gets up when he falls and keeps going. You cannot help your child find purpose until you have created the culture of drive in your home. Keep reading to discover some simple ways to apply all the lessons of drive.

Put Your Child in the Driver's Seat

Apply the Lessons of Drive

Uniting all the strategies is a message of hope for a positive future. Many kids have difficulty seeing past next week, let alone a decade from now. While it is important to live for today, we have to see how the choices we make will impact us later on. Kids need to understand that they will have an independent future—a unique life that will be lived individually, not in the shadow of their parents. They will have their own identity, purpose, friends, employment, hobbies, and spirit. Children with drive can see into the future with hope and optimism for a life that will be important and worth living. As you are working toward developing drive in your child (or young adult), it is critical that you apply each of the nine drive strategies in a way that moves this young human being to a state of individual identity, separate from yours.

Following is a recap of each of the nine lessons of drive and some additional simple applications for your own family.

1. Be a Pathfinder: Gather the Info That Really Makes a Difference

Really get to know your child in a way that is meaningful, without hovering like a helicopter. Pathfinder parents are not afraid to be the authority figure yet back off when the child needs more independence. Most important, a pathfinder parent ensures that a child takes responsibility for his or her own actions.

Middle school students

- Be sure to adequately supervise preteens and young teens. The most critical time of day is after school, before parents are home from work. This is when middle schoolers are most likely to get into all kinds of trouble that parents mistakenly believe only occurs with older children. Consider altering your schedules or work life so that somebody is home at this time.

- Rethink cell phone usage for this age group. If you do allow your child to have a cell phone, make sure he is using it to contact *you* at designated times. A middle schooler with a cell phone typically gets calls from his parent, who is checking in with him. It should be the other way around. Consider making your child do without the cell phone to drive this point home.

- Learn the lingo. Kids at this age frequently come up with their own language and enjoy entertainment that is completely foreign to their parents. Make it your business to become bilingual!

High school students

- Stop being a secretary for your teen. High school students should be able to order pizza, make medical appointments, fill out applications, and generally manage most of their own affairs. You will have to provide some guidance and instruction at first but will soon be able to stop providing administrative services. What a time-saver!

- Provide the keys, but not the car. Delaying the acquisition of a vehicle will help you keep better tabs on your almost grown teen.
- Avoid being one of the crowd. Many times parents are tempted to intervene in squabbles between a child and friends. Help your child figure out what to do, but avoid talking with the friend(s) and/or the parents of the friend(s) unless there is real danger of physical harm.

College students

- Feed the hungry. Be sure when you visit your child in college that you offer to take out one or two friends with you to a meal. Just watch and listen to get a good glimpse of how your child is adjusting to college. College kids are always hungry and will love this opportunity!
- Keep talking about drug and alcohol abuse all the way through college. Be careful of the assumption that all college kids experiment with drugs and alcohol with no long-term harm. Watch, listen, and pay close attention to signs that your college kid is overdoing the partying. Don't be afraid to confront and act if you believe there is a problem. Your child's life and future are at risk if you let this go unchecked.
- Move on with your life. This is a wonderful time when you can start doing some things for yourself. Don't wallow in the misery of missing your child; relish your newfound freedom to expand your horizons!

Young adults (who are not in college)

- Help your young adult continue to dream and explore. Travel together, and investigate anything and everything that might be of interest to him. Provide him with loads of opportunities for personal growth; after all, his education did not end with high school.

- Share your own plans for the future with your young adult. Be sure you are clear that your life is continuing and that you expect at some point he will move away from home.
- Take vacations without your grown child. Spend some time away to give both of you room to breathe. Just explain how the home should be run in your absence.

2. Increase Risk: Take Away the Plastic Bubble

Encourage your child to take chances. Your child cannot strive for success if he is forever fearful of failure. Teach him the value of failure and how to use it to grow and learn. Finding purpose involves taking a great deal of risk. It requires a person to put things on the line for what is truly important. Someone who is fearful of failing will not be able to move toward things that are meaningful.

Middle school students
- Find or create errands for your child to complete. Think of places within biking or ·walking distance from your home. Make your child responsible for handling dry cleaning, picking up a few groceries, or providing other services that will increase independence (and help lighten your load).
- Find safe places in nature for your child to explore. There is nothing like the feeling of exploring woodlands and other natural areas without adults around. Be sure he goes in a group, and provide guidance to keep them all safe. If there is nothing near your home, look for state or county parks. You can have a picnic with a friend while the kids go off into the wilderness.

- Provide home improvement projects for your child to tackle independently. Painting a bedroom, sewing new pillows or curtains, or other little projects are ideal. Keep in mind that the results are not going to be perfect. Just give your kids the room to take chances and learn from their mistakes.

High school students

- Let your child visit a sibling, cousin, or older friend who lives away at college. Talk about the risks involved and what your child can do to stay safe. This will provide a wonderful adventure and give your high school student some motivation to start thinking about the post-high-school years.
- Look for school or community activities that involve overnight travel, and have your high schooler participate in these activities—without you there. It will be great for your child and a break for you!
- Provide big-ticket fun for teens. Let them go to concerts or sporting events at stadiums. Let them take a train into a nearby city for the day with a plan in mind. Let them go and do and explore without you there.

College students

- Consider study abroad programs. Help your college kid explore the wonderful opportunities through these college programs.
- Provide a challenge. Encourage your college student to take difficult courses and to explore class options that require courage and risk.

Young adults (who are not in college)

- Help your young adult think outside the box of regular employment. You may have an entrepreneur who needs just a little encouragement. Help this young titan find funding and support for a new business endeavor.

- Is this the right place for your child to live? You may want to assist your adult child in moving to a brand-new city to try a different way of life.
- Sometimes work isn't all it's cracked up to be. Many young adults find themselves by traveling on a shoestring. They start with a little money and earn as they discover new lands. Encourage your child to think of places that might be fun to visit before getting saddled with financial obligations.

3. Decrease Rewards: Allow Life's Natural Consequences to Take Hold

If your child is rewarded regardless of effort on her part, she won't see much point in striving for more. Working and going to college tend to provide new perspectives in a person's life, allowing her to discover meaningful things. Someone who has everything given to her is likely to be content to slack or just stay home.

Middle school students
- Stop being the homework police. Provide the time and space for homework to get done, and then back off. Help your child make the connection between homework, grades, and other school consequences. Then allow the consequences to occur.
- Stop doing your child's laundry. This is a great way to drive the point of natural consequences home. Kids who don't do their laundry don't have clean clothes.
- Stop being your child's alarm clock. Transportation to school leaves at a designated time. Kids who miss it will have to make other arrangements.

High school students

- There are no free lunches. Require your teen to pay for school lunch out of the monthly budget you have established (see chapter 5) or to pack a lunch (using food you provide at home). If your teen is disorganized, lunch will cost more.

- Find natural consequences for behavior. If your teen speaks to you disrespectfully, don't respond. If your teen lies to you, require proof of her claims in future situations. If your teen is mean to someone, require service to others. If your teen doesn't get up on time, require an earlier bedtime. Try to avoid random "you're grounded" punishments, but instead help her connect behavior with consequences.

- Charge your teen for maid, chauffeur, and delivery service. If you choose to clean up your teen's bathroom, make an extra trip due to poor planning, or deliver a forgotten homework assignment, create an invoice that your teen must pay. Payment can be in cash or extra chores around the house.

College students

- Set up a meal plan and transportation plan and then send no money. If your college student runs out, don't send any more, except at the designated times you have established. Your college student will have to figure out how to make it until then. Of course, there may be true emergencies that require extra cash. Only in those situations should you step in and help.

- Help your college student see far into the future. Check out concert and special event schedules. If there is a big event coming up, ask your college student what can be done to get there. How much money is required? How can the budget be adjusted to allow for this additional expense? Will there need to be schedule adjustments to accommodate the event?

- Help your college student plan out her four years of school from the very beginning. Talk often about what will be required to reach her goals. Discuss grades each semester and what they mean in the context of her goals. If she gets off track, discuss ways to make things right.

Young adults (who are not in college)
- Continue to provide natural consequences. If your young adult and her friends eat all the food, lock it up and require your "boarder" to do her own grocery shopping. If you provide extra maid service, send a bill. If she abuses the computer, deny access.
- Continue to provide natural rewards. If your boarder provides extra services, reduce the rent. If she agrees to take on responsibilities—such as shuttling younger children, shopping, or running errands—provide the vehicle.
- Above all, don't bail out your young adult when she makes mistakes. Don't pay for her parking or speeding tickets, and don't give her money when she squanders her resources.

4. Deschedule: Encourage Joy, Imagination, and Creativity

If every single activity is scheduled, set, and structured, your child will not have a need to find things that are interesting and exciting. Most important, he will not have the time to imagine, create, and reflect. This kind of unstructured time is vital for him to develop the dreams that will lead him to true purpose and meaning in life.

Middle school students
- Create a daily schedule for your family and post it. Check and double-check that you have allowed enough unstructured time. Be careful not to infringe on others' free time.

- Play word games and tell stories. List several items that are seemingly unrelated, and ask your preteen to say a sentence that includes them all. Say a sentence to begin a story, and have your child say the next sentence. Keep going back and forth until you have a whole story.
- Draw together. Keep chalk on the front porch for the sidewalk. Cover your kitchen table with paper, and have crayons on hand.

High school students

Have a family conference at the beginning of each natural transition to a new school term or long break. Talk about the family routine and what you can do to keep enough unstructured time available.

- Allow your high schooler to sleep in on the weekends and just "be" from time to time.
- Continue to tell stories together. Talk about an actual event—and then exaggerate it to make it a real thriller.
- Get creative together. Decorate a room, plant a garden, or get involved in a project that will get your creative juices flowing.

College students

- Plan some weekend or vacation time together when you can kick back and relax.
- Be sure your college student has some downtime when she returns for school breaks. Understand that it is natural at this age for young adults to just be still for a short period following intense academic pressure.
- Take an interest in what she is learning each semester. If you listen long enough, you will learn about lots of things that have sparked her imagination.

Young adults (who are not in college)

- Continue to dream and imagine the future for your young adult. Ask questions like "What do you think you will be doing at my age?" If you two see someone who is obviously well off financially or really happy and content, talk about what that person does.
- Continue to explore leisure activities that allow for adventure and relaxation.
- Although you want to establish a family schedule, remember that everyone needs time without obligations or expectations from others.

5. Reduce Comfort: Counteract the Immense Abundance and Indulgence of Our Culture

If you provide a very comfortable home for your child, complete with all his favorite toys, he will not desire anything more. People who have everything handed to them are not likely to go out into the world in search of things. They already have everything they want. Reducing comfort creates desire, resulting in a young person gaining the experience and perspective that fuel purpose.

Middle school students

- Consider everything you give your preteen. Are they needs or wants? Think about gifts that might be appropriate for birthdays and holidays, and avoid buying things at other times. Make the birthdays and holidays truly special by reducing gift giving at other times.
- Engage your preteen in some strenuous tasks, like moving heavy boxes or pulling weeds. Encourage sweat whenever possible.

- Consider temporarily doing without some luxuries that your preteen may assume are automatically provided to everyone. Examples include air-conditioning, car entertainment systems, and televisions.

High school students
- Consider some rustic experiences, like camping, to provide some real examples of life without luxury.
- Go on a service vacation together, and do some hard work for others while enjoying less-than-luxurious accommodations.
- Consider a moratorium on shopping and spending for your family. Commit to a month or so without purchasing anything except the basics. Avoid going out to eat or paying for entertainment. This will provide a whole new perspective for your teen.

College students
- Consider your college student's living situation away from home. Ideally, it should be in a dorm with a roommate and shared bathroom facilities. This encourages new relationships and helps college students work cooperatively. As your student demonstrates success each year, you can provide better accommodations.
- Don't provide too much money for food, entertainment, books, and incidentals. Require that your college student get creative to control food and entertainment costs and investigate all options for obtaining required books and materials. As students demonstrate success academically, they can take on limited amounts of work for pay.
- When your college student comes home for breaks, be sure not to make things too wonderful. After all, you want her to go back to school!

Young adults (who are not in college)

- Look at the room or rooms that your adult child calls home. Have you provided too much space or luxury? Consider changing the accommodations so that you can have more space or things for yourself.
- Consider all that you do that makes life easier for your adult child and whether you should continue providing those services.
- Consider some of the luxuries that you provide, like cable television, gourmet coffee, and special cosmetics. If possible, reduce these to areas of the house that only you inhabit. Your adult child will have to pay for them or do without.

6. Delay Gratification: Resist the Quick Fixes of the Lottery, Game Shows, and Reality TV

Teach your child the true value of things by making him wait to earn them. Those who receive everything immediately learn impatience and ungratefulness.

Middle school students

- Help your preteen make the connection between studying and grades. This is an excellent example of delayed gratification. Kids have difficulty staying on track throughout a grading period without parental support. If your child needs more frequent feedback, consider getting grade updates from the teacher each week so you can guide your middle schooler. Gradually decrease the weekly reminders until your child can stay on track consistently.
- Think about a family "want," such as a new television. Together with your preteen, create a family plan to save money by doing without things so you can purchase the television.

- Plan a family trip to a theme park. Assist your preteen in saving up money ahead of time so that he can purchase extra things like special admissions to attractions.

High school students
- Plan a family vacation, and talk about all that must happen leading up to the event. Develop a timeline of all the tasks involved, like updating passports, making kennel reservations, buying clothes for the trip, and so on. Create a budget, and determine where the family will get the needed money. Engage your teen in the planning process by assigning tasks. Meet each week to check on progress, and help connect the tasks to the event.
- Talk about post-high-school goals, and establish a timeline of things that must happen to reach those goals.
- Use the normal events in high school, like formal dances and sporting events, to motivate your teen. Again, talk about all that must happen for him to participate, and be sure that everything is completed on time.

College students
- The very nature of college is to delay gratification. Talk often about the purpose of a good education and why it is important to persevere.
- Encourage your college student to enjoy this wonderful time of discovery and fun. Although some students may be anxious while they are waiting to begin their life, be sure to convey the message that life is indeed happening in college!
- Your college student may see working people who are his age and become envious. He may believe that he is wasting his time in school while others are making money. Talk about finding that balance. Share research that confirms that college

graduates earn more throughout life than their counterparts who have not completed college.

Young adults (who are not in college)
- Young adults must continue to look toward the future and set goals. Keep this dialogue open at all times.
- The difference between a dream and a goal is a timeline. Be a life coach to your child. Have a monthly meeting when you go out to dinner together to review the timeline and stay on track.
- Celebrate successes! Every time your young adult takes a step toward a goal, be sure to make a big deal out of it. Do something fun together to make the event special.

7. Encourage Accomplishment: Create a Sense of Self through True Achievement

Someone who is rewarded for things that are not real achievements may already believe that he has succeeded and will have no desire to accomplish other things. It is vital to find ways to encourage true accomplishment—especially for your young adult still living at home.

Middle school students
- Provide opportunities for accomplishment at home. Consider your child's accomplishment when he completes each task. Avoid just commenting on or rewarding effort. Communicate to your preteen how well he accomplished a task.
- If your middle schooler comes home with a bad grade, discuss what he could have done to alter the result. If the child talks about an unfair teacher or task, don't accept that as an excuse. Instead, ask what the *child* could have done differently to meet the teacher's expectations, even if those expectations were unfair.

- Avoid language like "good job" and "way to go" when the child really has not succeeded. Instead, provide caring, honest feedback that focuses on what he can learn from the experience and how he can improve the level of accomplishment next time.

High school students

- Share stories of your own successes and failures and what caused each. Ask your teen to share similar stories. Together identify what makes someone succeed or fail.
- Talk about some project or undertaking in your current life and what it will take to succeed. Ask your teen for advice on what might increase your chances of success, and talk about the worst thing that might happen if you fail. Be sure to point out that you are still the same person, regardless of whether you succeed or fail.
- Talk about your high schooler's perception of a successful peer. Help distinguish between popular people and those who have truly accomplished things.

College students and young adults

- Really pay attention to your college student or young adult's small accomplishments as he is seeking and exploring. Earning a good grade, receiving a small raise, gaining insight into the future, and saving enough for a car are all examples of accomplishments. Be sure to recognize when he has achieved these things, and let him know that you noticed.
- Really celebrate the big accomplishments, like passing a very challenging class, getting a new job, or getting accepted into an internship or school.
- Always remember that failure brings new insights, and help your adult child learn from mistakes and move on with a healthy self-concept.

8. Control the Crowd: Use Peers for Positive Influence and Independence

Be sure your child is choosing friends who will create a positive influence. They should be people who want things in life and understand what it takes to get them. A driven person usually surrounds himself with others who are driven.

Middle school students
- Encourage your preteen and friends to set some goals together. They can lean on each other when things get tough. This might include joining a sports team together or studying for a challenging class.
- Provide events for this positive peer group to work and socialize together. Encourage this healthy support group.
- Use this process to reduce the time your preteen spends with nondriven friends (whom you have identified using the strategies listed in chapter 10) and to increase his time with more driven peers.

High school students
- Be an uncool listener. Always listen to what your teen and friends have to say, but provide a voice of maturity and reason when you have a chance to contribute to the conversation.
- Be a fly on the wall when you are playing chauffeur or party host. Really understand what this peer group is all about so you can act when necessary.
- Continually confront your teen about friends who are not headed in the right direction. Don't be afraid to say things that your teen may perceive as negative. Do whatever you can to increase her time with driven friends and decrease her time with ones who are not driven.

College students

- If your college student is interested in joining a sorority or fraternity, make it your business to learn about each organization he or she is considering. You should be able to get stats like grade point averages, graduation rates, and success rates for each. Allow your college student to only pledge the groups that meet your standards. You have a lot of control here. Greek organizations are generally very expensive. Your college student will probably require your assistance (and your approval) to participate.

- Don't pressure your college student to rush into selecting a major to prepare for a career, unless he is already passionate about a particular field. Instead, encourage him to focus on taking courses that will include driven students. For example, a certain major at a university may have the reputation of being easy. Encourage your college student to take introductory courses in majors that are known to attract more driven students.

- Talk to your college student about where his friends from high school are. Discuss which ones were driven in high school and how they are doing versus the ones who may have been less motivated. There may be friends who were not driven then but are now. Talk about what caused the change in these students. Use his old friends as examples of the benefits of developing drive.

Young adults (who are not in college)

- The time period immediately following high school can be a very difficult time for young adults who have not gone to college or young adults who have quickly returned home after a bad college experience. You will need to be very aware of your adult child's friends and their powerful influences. Check out your adult child's social-networking Web sites to understand her current peer group. Look for arrested development. If all your young adult's friends are interested in things that resemble interests of high school students, you may have a problem. Talk about where friends are going with their lives and other potential peer groups. Continue discussing why it is important to surround oneself with positive people.

- Remember what things you can control, and use that power to decrease your adult child's access to negative friends. Use the car keys, availability of your home to guests, money, and any other things that you control to move your young adult in the right direction.

- Try and find some people at work, or through friends, who are just a little older and may have interests similar to your adult child's. Invite them to your home for dinner and see whether you can help your young adult find some new peers close to home who are a bit further along in their development.

9. Create a Sense of Purpose: Make Life Meaningful

To help your child find purpose, you need to know what he thinks and feels. Find those things that are important to him and expand them. Do all you can to open your child up to life's possibilities!

Middle school students
- Establish a short list of family values that will become the filter through which decisions are made. For example, in our home, we valued honesty and kindness above all else. These became the filter through which our children had to process each behavioral decision they made.

- Help your middle schooler develop a personal set of values that will include activities or things that she values above all others. This should be a longer list than your family values. Have your preteen create a poster to hang in her bedroom or the kitchen as a reminder.
- Talk with your preteen about your personal values and how they guide your decisions. Have a continual dialogue about what is important to each member of the family and how you all support each others' values and balance what may be conflicting priorities.

High school students and beyond
- Review your teen or young adult's personal values once or twice each year, or more often if necessary. Talk about an appropriate selection of activities to support her personal values and what activities may conflict with them.
- Link your teen or young adult's personal values to college and career exploration. What colleges or educational opportunities support these values? What jobs and careers would be linked to them? Use her personal values to explore a wide variety of options.
- Talk with your teen or young adult about how each decision supports or conflicts with values. Use them to guide your discussions about friends, activities, course selections, choice of majors, choice of jobs and careers, places of worship, and all other things in her life.
- Celebrate the "a-ha" moments that will inevitably come. Don't be passé when your teen or young adult tells you of a great personal insight or discovery that involves finding one's place in the world. Accept it for the amazing epiphany that it is (even if you believe it may change later), and use it to help you help your child propel her life forward.

Overall Strategies for Developing Drive

As your child grows and learns, create a culture of drive in your home. Here are some final tips to help you do this.

- Steer your child in the right direction without hovering.
- Encourage your child to take chances.
- Allow your child to experience negative consequences caused by his behavior.
- Get rid of electronics in the bedroom, in the car, and at the table.
- Have dinner as a family as much as possible.
- Make mornings less stressful. Keep the TV and radio off, and talk to your children.
- Require your child to try one new sport and one new arts activity each year.
- Require your children to finish everything they start—never let them quit unless there is real danger.
- Find a school that will support your goals for your child—think about learning styles and homework load.
- Find time to be with your child, particularly as he becomes an adolescent.
- Balance your family life and your child's life with plenty of quality time together and time when there isn't anything in particular to do.
- Stay connected to your children in meaningful ways. Really know them as people, and know their friends.
- Connect your child to the world through friends, travel, reading, and research.
- Allow your child to win and lose gracefully.
- Allow your child to experience failure and learn from it.
- Praise and reward only true accomplishments.

- Provide your child with opportunities to be important to others and to give.
- Don't be afraid to be the parent. You are not doing your child any favors by being a friend.

Driven People Drive Our World

Think about people in your community who really make a positive difference. Is there a teacher who takes special interest in children and will work tirelessly to help them succeed? Is there a business leader who organizes others to improve infrastructure in your town? Is there a politician who is concerned for local citizens and champions laws to improve others' lives? Have you enjoyed the talents of an amazing musician who moved you with a performance? Do you appreciate the beauty of incredible architecture? People who improve our communities, lead our world, and provide us with art and beauty are driven. They want to be things—to do things—to engage in life in a meaningful way. Help your child lead an exciting life full of promise that improves the lives of others. Everything is possible with drive.

Index

abundance in modern American life, 15–17. *See also* comforts, value of reducing
academic load during college years, 120
accomplishments, encouraging, 141–158
  alternatives to trophy culture and, 157–159
  during college years, 207
  competition as means of, 144–145, 151
  during high school years, 153–154, 207
  during middle school years, 152–153, 206–207
  self-esteem and, 143–144
  winning and, 145–148
  during young adult years, 154–157, 207
activities, overscheduled. *See* descheduling
Admissions, 111–112
adult children. *See* young adult years

afterschool activities, 67
alcohol use
  during college years, 195
  hot air balloon parents and, 37
  and parenting skills generally, 44–48
allowances, 85
American Idol, 17, 127, 135
American life, realities of modern. *See* modern American life, realities of
apathy during high school years, 84–86
Apple, 94
arrests, 159–160
arts, 67–68
attendance at school, 82
attention, need for, 76

baby boomers, 6
balance, living in, 105–108
battles, choosing, 80
behavioral science, 71–72
behaviors, improving children's, 74–75

best friends, parents as, 171–174
Boys Town, 79
butterfly years, 68–69

calm environments, providing,
    100
camps, 170
cars
    during college years, 121
    as comfort zones, 112
    desire to drive, 3
    during high school years,
        65–66, 84–85, 195
    teenagers and, 16–17
caterpillar years, 61–64
cell phones. *See also* technology
    during college years, 51–52
    in goal-setting, 133
    during middle school years,
        194
    during teenage years,
        117–118
    during young adult years, 125
Center for Generational Studies, 4
change, dealing with, 27
chaperoning events, 49–50
charitable giving, 185–188
cheating, 157
checking accounts, 51
chores, 80–81
Christmas, 187
chrysalis years, 64–68
cigarettes, 45
cleanliness, 115
clothing, giving away, 186
coaches, 147–148
college education
    accomplishments during,
        155–157, 207
    goals of, 133–134
    planning for, 200

college years
    comforts during, 118–122, 203
    descheduling, 201
    dos and don'ts for parents
        during, 50–52
    drive questionnaire for, 30–32
    gratification during, 205–206
    pathfinder parenting during,
        195
    peers during, 209
    rewards during, 198–200
    risks during, 197
    underachievement during,
        86–87
comforts, value of reducing,
    109–126
    during adult years, 122–126
    during college years, 118–122,
        203
    family vehicles as comfort
        zones, 112
    during high school years,
        116–118, 203
    during middle school years,
        113–116, 202–203
    potty training and, 110–111
    strollers, influence of, 111–112
    during young adult years, 204
community service projects,
    186–187
competition, 141–158
    goals of, 148–151
    healthy, 158
    during high school years,
        153–154
    importance of, 144–145
    during middle school years,
        152–153
    self-esteem, building, 143–144
    winning, desire for, 145–148
computer use, 48–49

consequences, 12–14, 52–53.
    See also rewards, value of
    decreasing
control issues, 78–79
Cosby, Bill, 11
costs of living, 86
couch use, 105
creating drive, 19–22
creativity, encouraging. *See*
    descheduling
credit cards, 51
cultural events, 199, 205
culture, 191–192
cursing, 83
cyberrelationships, 42, 48–49

A Dating Story, 122
decision-making skills, 102, 104
defiance during middle school
    years, 80–84
dependency, 10–11
deprogrammed children, 99
descheduling, 91–108
    balance of life and, 105–108
    calm environments, providing,
        100
    during college years, 201
    deprogrammed children, 99
    group activities for, 102
    during high school years,
        102–104, 201
    during middle school years,
        100–102, 200–201
    need for, 14–15
    nutrition and, 101
    outdoor exercise in, 101
    overscheduling activities vs.,
        92–95
    programming defined, 95–99
    structured activities vs. free
        time, 100

tomorrow, preparing for,
    100–101
during young adult years, 202
desire
    drive vs., 24–26
    for fame, 129–130
    to win, 145–148
diapers, 111
directionless high school students,
    116–118
distractible middle schoolers,
    100–102
dorm living, 203
dos and don'ts during college
    years, 50–52
driver's seat, putting children in,
    193–213
    accomplishments, encouraging,
        206–207
    during college years, 195
    comforts, reducing, 202–204
    descheduling, 200–202
    gratification, delaying, 204–206
    during high school years,
        194–195
    during middle school years,
        194
    pathfinder parents and,
        194–196
    peers, positive influence of,
        208–210
    purpose, creating sense of,
        210–211
    rewards, decreasing, 198–200
    risks, increasing, 196–198
    during young adult years,
        195–196
driving
    license for, 65–66
    as reward, 84–85
    under the influence, 159–160

dropout rates, 116
drug and alcohol use
    during college years, 195
    hot air balloon parents and, 37
    parenting skills generally,
        44–48
drunk driving, 159–160

elementary school years, 61–64
Elkind, Dr. David, 15, 93
encouragement. *See* accomplish-
    ments, encouraging
errands, 196
exercise
    during high school years, 104
    during middle school years, 101
    outdoor, 146
Extreme Makeover, 127
extrinsic motivators, 72
eye rolling, 83

F.B.I.'s Uniform Crime Report of
    2004, 5
fame, desire for, 129–130
family conferences, 201
fashion, 62
finishing tasks, 27
Florida State University (FSU),
    134
fraternities, 209
free time vs. structured activities,
    100
fresh air and exercise, 101, 104
friends, influence of, 159–174
    befriending children's friends,
        164–165
    parenting vs. friendship,
        171–174
    quality of, 162–164
    questions to ask, 50, 165–168
    redirecting choices, 168–170

future, children's vision of, 85–86,
    118
future for children
    abundance influencing, 15–17
    dependency and, 10–11
    Generation Me, 3–8
    immediate gratification and,
        17–18
    in modern American life, 10,
        19–22
    overscheduled activities and,
        14–15
    plastic bubble in, 11–12
    rewards without consequences,
        12–14
    success in, 8–10
    underachievement influencing,
        18–19

game shows, 204–206
games, playing, 146
Generation Gap, 6
Generation Me, 3–8
*Generation Me: Why Today's Young
    Americans Are More Confi-
    dent, Assertive, Entitled—
    and More Miserable Than
    Ever Before*, 16
Generation X, 6–7
Generation Y. *See* Generation Me
gift giving, 202
giving to charity, 185–188
goals
    of competitive participation,
        148–151
    defined, 128
    during high school years,
        133–135, 205
    during middle school years,
        132–133
God, relationship to, 189–191

Google, 94
grades
    during college years, 86, 156
    during high school years, 85, 86
    during middle school years,
        204, 206
    rewards and, 81–82
graduation ceremonies, 141–142
gratification, value of delaying,
        127–139
    during college years, 205–206
    fame and, 129–130
    during high school years,
        133–135, 205
    instant American culture vs.,
        130
    during middle school years,
        132–133, 204–205
    modern American life vs., 17–18
    money and, 135–139
    results, earning, 129
    visualization of goals, 130–132
    during young adult years, 206
Greek organizations, 209
group activities, 102
guests
    listening to, 50, 163, 165
    during young adult years,
        124–125

hair styles, 62
Hanukkah, 187
head tossing, 83
helicopter parents
    activities, scheduling, 98
    parenting skills of, 36–37, 40
high school years
    accomplishments during,
        153–154, 207
    apathy during, 84–86
    comforts during, 116–118, 203

descheduling, 102–104, 201
drive questionnaire for, 28–29
gratification during, 205
long-term goals, 133–135
pathfinder parenting during,
    194–195
peers during, 208
purpose during, 211
questions for friends during,
    166–167
rewards during, 84–86, 199
risks during, 64–68, 197
holiday giving, 187
home improvement projects, 197
homesickness during college years,
    121–122
homework, 198
hot air balloon parents
    activities, scheduling, 98
    parenting skills of, 37–38,
        40–41
house schedules, 105
household chores
    during high school years, 85,
        117
    during middle school years,
        80–81, 83
    during young adult years, 105,
        124
hovering vs. involvement, 44

imagination, encouraging. See
    descheduling
immediate gratification, 17–18.
    See also gratification, value of
    delaying
independent thinking, 102, 104
indulgence, counteracting. See
    comforts, value of reducing
instant American culture, 130
insults, 83

intervention levels, 52–53, 208
intrinsic motivators, 72
involvement vs. hovering, 44

jaded young adults, 104–105
jobs
    class time as interview for, 155
    opportunities for, 197–198
    placement services, 155
    for teens, 66–67
    training for, 154–155
joint checking accounts, 51
joy, encouraging. *See* descheduling

kicking young adults out of the
    house, 125

laundry
    during middle school years, 80,
        114, 198
    during young adult years, 124
liberal arts education, purpose of,
    155–156
Lieberman, Nancy, 111
life quality, 28
life realities in modern America.
        See modern American life,
        realities of
lingo, learning, 194
listening
    during college years, 195
    to friends, 49–50
    during high school years, 208
long-term goals, 133–135
losing, lessons of, 146, 153–154
lotteries, 204–206
lunch money, 199–200
luxuries, doing without, 203–204

major selection in college, 209
Maslow, Abraham, 176–177

the matures, 6
meal plans, 51–52, 199
meals with family, 105
Microsoft, 94
middle school years
    accomplishments during,
        152–153, 206–207
    comforts during, 113–116,
        202–203
    defiance during, 80–84
    descheduling, 200–201
    drive questionnaire for, 28–29
    gratification during, 204–205
    pathfinder parenting during,
        194–196
    peers, positive influence of, 208
    purpose, creating sense of,
        210–211
    questions for friends during,
        165–166
    rewards, value of decreasing,
        80–84, 198
    risks during, 61–64, 196–197
    short-term goals, 132–133
millennial generation. *See*
        Generation Me
modern American life, realities of,
        10–22
    abundance, 15–17
    dependency, 10–11
    drive, learning, 19–22
    immediate gratification, 17–18
    overscheduled activities, 14–15
    plastic bubble in, 11–12
    rewards without consequences,
        12–14
    underachievement, 18–19
money
    allowances, 85
    earning, 27
    lunch, 199–200

rent, 125, 200
saving, 204–205
value of, 135–139
moocher adult children, 87–89
morning home environments, 103
motivation, testing, 23–33
  defining drive, 26–28
  drive vs. desire, 24–26
  questionnaires for, 28–33

name-calling, 83
nature, exploring, 196
NISMART report of 2005, 61
Now and Then, 59
nutrition
  in balanced living, 96
  for behavior change, 74
  during high school years,
    103–104
  during middle school years, 101

Odyssey of the Mind, 102
one-on-one attention, 77–78
outdoor exercise, 104, 146
overscheduled activities, 14–15

parasitic adult children, 122–126
parenting skills, 35–55
  alcohol use, 44–48
  chaperoning events, 49–50
  college students, dos and don'ts
    for, 50–52
  computer use, 48–49
  drug use, 44–48
  friends, asking about, 50
  of helicopter parents, 36–37, 40
  of hot air balloon parents,
    37–38, 40–41
  intervention levels, 52–53
  introduction to, 35–36
  involvement vs. hovering, 44

of pathfinder parents, 38–39,
    41–43
  relationships with children,
    53–55
  schools, relationship with, 49
  smoking, signs of, 45
  social time, listening during,
    50
  stealth reconnaissance, 43–44
  whereabouts of children,
    knowing, 44
parenting vs. friendship, 171–174
pathfinder parents
  activities and, 98–99
  consequences and, 52–53
  parenting skills of, 38–39,
    41–43
Pavlov, Ivan, 71–72
payment for services, 199, 200
Peale, Norman Vincent, 131
peers, positive influence of,
    159–174
  befriending children's friends,
    164–165
  during college years, 209
  during high school years, 195,
    208
  during middle school years,
    208
  parenting vs. friendship,
    171–174
  quality of friends, influencing,
    162–164, 168–170
  questions to ask friends,
    165–168
  during young adult years,
    209–210
Pelley, Scott, 9–10
performing arts, 67–68
personal belongings, giving away,
    186

physiological needs, 79–80
plastic bubble, 11–12, 59–61. *See also* risks, value of increasing
"Pomp and Circumstance," 141
positive thinking, 130–131
post high school years, 68–69, 167–168. *See also* college years
potty training, 110–111
Pour Your Heart into It, 8
power balance, 75–76
The Power of Play, 93
The Power of Positive Thinking, 130–131
privilege vs. ownership, 118
public transportation, 51
punishments, 82–83
purpose, creating sense of, 175–192
    attributes of, 183–185
    connections for, 188–189
    culture and, 191–192
    defined, 178–183
    giving for, 185–188
    during high school years and beyond, 211
    during middle school years, 210–211
    spirituality for, 189–191
The Purpose-Driven Life, 178
pyramid of basic needs, 177

questionnaires for testing motivation, 28–33
questions to ask friends, 165–168
quitting, advising against, 152

rating scale, for drive questionnaires, 32
realistic self-sense, 144
reality TV shows, 17, 204–206
reconnaissance. *See* stealth reconnaissance
reducing comforts, value of. *See* comforts, value of reducing
relationship skills, 4, 27
relevance, 185
religious practice, 189–191
Renaissance Academy, 19–21
rent, 125, 200
respect, demanding, 83–84, 199
responsibility, giving, 80–81
results, earning, 129
rewards, value of decreasing, 71–89
    age factors, 80
    allowances, 85
    appropriate rewards, 82
    attention, need for, 76
    behaviors, improving children's, 74–75
    during college years, 86–87, 198–200
    control issues, 78–79
    costs of living and, 86
    driving, 84–85
    future vision and, 85–86
    grades and, 81
    during high school years, 84–86, 199
    during middle school years, 80–84, 198
    in modern American life, 12–14
    during moocher adult years, 87–89
    one-on-one attention, providing, 77–78
    physiological needs, 79–80
    power balance in, 75–76
    punishments vs., 82–83
    respect, demanding, 83–84

technology, limiting, 78
transitions, school to home,
    76–77
during young adult years,
    200
risks, value of increasing, 57–70
    during college years, 197
    driver's seat, putting children
        in, 196–198
    during elementary and middle
        school years, 61–64
    example of, 69–70
    during high school years,
        64–68, 197
    during middle school years,
        61–64, 196–197
    plastic bubble, preventing,
        59–61
    during post high school years,
        68–69
    during young adult years,
        197–198
role models, other adults as, 189
Rosa, Jan, 79

The Sandlot, 59
saving money, 204–205
schedules, 14–15, 106–107.
    See also descheduling
school of drive, 19–22
schools
    grades in. See grades
    online services of, 51
    parent's relationships to, 49
Schultz, Howard, 8–10
screen time, limiting, 102
The Secret, 130–131
secretaries, parents as, 194–195
secretiveness, 43
self-actualization, 176–177
self-esteem, building, 143–144

self-sense, creating via achieve-
    ment. See accomplishments,
    encouraging
Serenity Prayer for Parents, 53
short-term goals, 132–133
60 Minutes, 9–10
Skinner, B. F., 71–72
slow-track college students,
    118–122
smoking, 45
social time, listening during, 50
social-networking sites, 48–49,
    209
SODAS method, 79
sororities, 209
speeding tickets, 200
spelling bees, 144
spending habits, 51
spirituality, 189–191
Spock, Dr. Benjamin, 12
Stand By Me, 59
stealth reconnaissance, 43–55
    chaperoning events, 49–50
    college students, dos and
        don'ts, 50–52
    computer use, 48–49
    drug and alcohol use, 44–48
    friends, asking about, 50
    intervention levels, 52–53
    involvement vs. hovering, 44
    reconnecting with children,
        53–55
    at school, 49
    smoking, signs of, 45
    social time, listening during, 50
    whereabouts of children and,
        44
stimuli, limiting, 100
stool refusal, 111
strategies for drive development,
    212–213

strenuous tasks, 202

strollers, 111–112

structured activities vs. free time,
100–102

substance abuse. *See* drug and
alcohol use

sugar consumption, 101, 103

summer vacations. *See* vacations

supervision, 194

technology. *See also* cell phones
computer use, 48–49
cyberrelationships, 42
Generation Me using, 4
in goal-setting, 132–133
intrusion of, 10–11
rewards and, 78
during young adult years, 125

testing motivation. *See* motivation,
testing

Thanksgiving, 187

A Theory of Human Motivation,
176

thinking, power of, 130–131

tomorrow, preparing for, 100–101

transitions, school to home,
76–77

transportation
during college years, 121, 199
during high school years,
117–118
during middle school years,
114
during young adult years,
124

travel
during college years, 197
during high school years, 170,
197
during young adult years,
195–196

trophy culture, 142–143,
157–159

Twenge, Dr. Jean, 16

uncertainty, dealing with, 27

underachievement, 18–19, 86–87

unmet physiological needs, 79–80

unmotivated middle schoolers,
113–116

U.S. Department of Justice, 5, 61

vacations
during college years, 201
culture during, 191
during high school years, 203,
205
summer, 66
without young adult children,
196

values, 179–183, 210–211. *See also*
purpose, creating sense of

visualization of goals, 130–132

vocational school, 154–155

volunteering
as charitable giving, 185–188
during high school years,
66–67, 153

waking up
during college years, 52
descheduling, 103, 105
during middle school years,
198

Walker, Howard, 53–54

walking away, 84

Warren, Rick, 178

What Not to Wear, 122–123

whereabouts of children, knowing,
44

White, Shaun, 69–70

winning, desire for, 145–148

word games, 201
work during college years, 121
work satisfaction, 27

yelling vs. constructive coaching,
    147–148
young adult years
  accomplishments during,
    154–157, 207
  comforts during, 122–126, 204
  descheduling, 104–105, 202
  gratification during, 206
  pathfinder parenting of,
    195–196
  peers during, 209–210
  rewards during, 200
  risks during, 197–198